Over The
Water Fall

Marilyn Martone, Ph.D.

Dedication

This book is dedicated to all those who made this story possible.

Table of Contents

$7.22

Acknowledgments

It is impossible to acknowledge individually all who were part of this story. Yet each played a major role in nurturing Michelle back to life. Without her family, especially her father and brothers Nick, Larry, and Tim, this story would have had a much different ending. I also wish to thank Carol DiPaolo, Genie Masterson, and Jane Rosenman for their editorial help as well as Elizabeth Kaplan who believed in this book when so many others did not.

Mostly, my thanks to Michelle, who continues to bring joy and meaning to our daily lives.

Introduction

Most of us have some idea of how we would like to live our lives. There are always setbacks along the way and sometimes, pleasant surprises but there is usually a general direction to our journey of life.

My life was typical of many women who came of age in the sixties. I went to college, worked for a few years and then got married and started a family. After several years of full-time homemaking and four children, I knew I needed more and decided to go back to school. I was a language major as an undergraduate but I did not want to further my formal education in languages because I loved languages in order to speak to other people not to read literature. When I sent off for my college transcript I noticed that philosophy and theology were always my strongest subjects. I also thought that our scientific developments had far outpaced our ethical understanding of those issues so I decided to pursue a masters' degree in health-care ethics. When my masters' degree was completed I still had many more pressing questions so I continued my studies and received a doctoral degree in moral theology. I pursued these degrees for the sake of knowledge and earned a full-time teaching position in theology. I loved teaching but I never had working as a full-time professor as my main goal in life.

Several years after I began teaching, my life took a dramatic turn and I came to understand the real reason why I had earned a Ph.D. The knowledge, the research skills, the contacts, and the credentials were all put in place in order to prepare me to undertake the greatest challenge of my life – to help save my daughter's life.

Theology has often been defined as "faith seeking understanding" and I brought my training as a theologian to my daughter's bedside. As her mother I did what mothers do but as a theologian I needed to find meaning in this event. I was not interested in negating it or putting a cheerful spin on it or even coping with it. I wanted to know what possible meaning I could find. So I did what academics do. I turned to books. The story gave rise to questions that needed answers. Reading taught me that I was not alone in this tragedy. On the written page I found solace and connection in the words of others.

What follows is an account of this story, a story that is still continuing. It shows how a theologian, an ethicist, and a mother used all her skills in order to stand by and protect her daughter and give meaning to both their lives when most of society had given up on them.

1.

The Phone Call

The phone call arrived about 7:30 pm on February 22, 1998. It was a cold, rainy Sunday evening, and my husband, Larry, and I had just returned from an afternoon with friends. Larry was in the den watching TV, and I was preparing to take a bath. As I passed the den, I saw him holding the phone to his ear and noticed a puzzled look on his face. Then I heard him say, "Michelle?"

Immediately, I stopped and began to feel my heart pounding. Who's calling about Michelle? Michelle is our twenty-one year old daughter, who is a fourth-year student at the University of Chicago. We had just spoken to her that morning, and she told us that she was spending the day writing a paper and cleaning her room. Who could be calling about Michelle?

Then I heard Larry say, "You'll have to talk to my wife," and he passed the phone to me.

The man whose voice I heard on the other end introduced himself as Dr. Wayne from Cook County Hospital in Chicago. He told me that Michelle had been hit by a car. She had suffered severe brain trauma and was on a ventilator. Hospital staff was preparing to rush Michelle into brain surgery. Although he continued and said that she had no other internal injuries, my mind was stuck on two words: *brain* and *ventilator*. I teach health-care ethics, and I knew that when these two words are used in the same sentence it's very serious. But this was not a classroom discussion – we were talking about my daughter. Somehow, I was able to write down the doctor's name and the name and phone number of the hospital before I hung up.

I had always feared receiving a phone call like this. I remember, when the children were young, every time I heard the alarm sound off from the firehouse for an ambulance call, I would take mental inventory as to where my children were and would be startled at the sound of the phone ringing soon after the alarm sounded. And now, the dreaded phone call had arrived. It was no longer a possibility but a fact. My daughter had been hit by a car and was dying, and we were a thousand miles away. For many years, I had worried about what I would do if something like this happened, and now I was about to find out.

Somehow my brain went into overdrive. Although my body was numb, I began to calculate in a very systematic order what needed to be done. I called my other children, all sons in their twenties, who lived in an apartment nearby. Tim was the only one I was able to reach. I asked him to find us a flight to Chicago while I contacted my sister, Kathie, who lives in Pennsylvania, and asked her to notify my family. Then I called my mother-in-law. I was hoping Mama would not answer the phone and that I could give the message to someone else. The day before, my father-in-law had had a massive stroke and was in the local hospital in intensive care, and I wasn't sure how much stress Mama could stand. She did answer the phone, but fortunately there were several other family members with her.

Now that our families were notified, we began preparing to leave for Chicago. I remember thinking that I would be spending a great deal of time in waiting rooms and that I should pack only sweat suits and sneakers, knowing they'd be comfortable to sleep in. My daughter was dying, and I was thinking about packing clothes that would be comfortable.

As we were finishing our packing, Tim arrived, telling us he was able to book us on a 9 pm flight out of La Guardia Airport in New York to Chicago's O'Hare. Soon after that, my sister-in-law Rose and our cousin Laurie arrived. The phone began to ring. My sister-in-law Donna asked what she could do. I told her to contact my friends. Michelle's boyfriend, Chris, called. Others from Chicago began to call, but I just wanted to get out of the house and get to my daughter. Rose took over the phone lines while Laurie, Larry, Tim, and I prepared to begin the half-hour drive to La Guardia.

I looked at the clock. It was 7:55. It was a Sunday night, about the time that the traffic is heaviest on the Long Island Expressway. Everyone was returning to the city after the weekend. Would we get to the airport on time? We had to. I had to get to my daughter as fast as possible. Was she still alive? How was the surgery going? What would I do if she died? Laurie told me that as I was getting into the car I said, "Now I will know if my faith holds up," although I don't remember much of what I said during that time. I do remember feeling, however, that this was the big one. This was the test of a lifetime.

We got into Laurie's car, although Tim drove. I sat numb in the back seat, worried that we wouldn't get to the airport on time, calculating how we would inform our other two sons, thinking about how to coordinate information on Michelle, pondering who else needed to be called. So many details. Laurie sat next to me taking notes. The cat! I had forgotten the cat. Fortunately, Laurie hadn't. I had given her the key to the house, and she told me she'd take care of the cat.

My mind was racing. I'd call from the airport and ask my friends Don and Julie to go to our sons' apartment later that evening to tell Nick and Larry what had happened. I didn't want to leave this message on their answering machine. I wanted someone to be with them when they heard the news. Did they have enough money for the plane tickets? I hoped their credit cards weren't maxed out.

Work! I was supposed to be back at work tomorrow. This was the last day of our week's winter vacation and I was supposed to be in the classroom tomorrow. I turned to Laurie and she scribbled in her notebook, "Call Father Ruiz first thing in the morning." Who else, who else? Joan. Call Joan. Joan is the mother of Michelle's good friend, Tamara, and she probably wouldn't get the phone call as part of the chain that Donna would initiate. But Joan and her husband, Arnie, needed to know. Michelle was like their daughter. In fact, Michelle called them, "Mommy 2" and "Daddy 2." Arnie was also Michelle's primary-care physician. Laurie wrote down, "Call Joan."

I wondered how I was going to keep everyone informed once I arrived in Chicago. I couldn't keep calling everyone. I needed a point person – one person who I could call and who would relay the messages. It couldn't be my mother-in-law. She would be busy with Pop. Everyone was so busy. Who would be home? Laurie turned to me and said, "Why not my mom?" Perfect. Because of a health condition, Aunt Noreen is always home. She's cool headed. She's methodical. She would take good notes, and I've always felt very close to her. It was decided. I would call Aunt Noreen, and she would pass the messages on.

I looked at my watch. It was 8:15. I worried about whether we would arrive at the airport in time. Fortunately, there wasn't much traffic on the road, but one could never tell. The next minute might find us caught in a traffic jam.

At 8:25, we pulled up in front of the American Airlines terminal at La Guardia Airport. We jumped out of the car. Laurie returned to the driver's seat while the rest of us went rushing to the tickets desk of American Airlines. Yes, they were expecting us. We informed them that this was a medical emergency, and we were able to get special rate tickets. Then we went to the designated gate and boarded the plane. As I got on the plane, I said to the flight attendant who was standing by the door, "I need you to know that I'm in shock." How ridiculous that must have sounded. But I knew that something was wrong with me because I had no feelings and I didn't know how it would play out. I thought I needed someone to know that if I started to act up on the plane there was a reason.

As we entered the plane, we saw that there were very few people on board. We went to our seats, and soon after we settled in, Tim's cell phone rang. It was my sister asking if we had any more news. We told her we were on a plane waiting for take off to Chicago. The flight attendant saw us using a cell phone, and we had to get off the plane and stand outside the plane door to finish our conversation. After the call, we went back to our seats and right before take off our son Larry came running down the aisle. When he returned home from work, he found a message on his answering machine from his cousin Paul, who told him of Michelle's accident. He then called our house, and my sister-in-law Rose told him we were on a 9 pm American Airlines flight out of LaGuardia. Without thinking, he ran to his car and drove to La Guardia. It was February, but he had no coat, no suitcase. When he heard the news, he just ran to his car, drove to the airport, parked the car, and ran to the plane, hoping to find us.

Soon, the plane took off, and we were on our way to Chicago. We all just sat in silence, lost in our own thoughts. Could this really be happening? I thought about Michelle. From the day of her birth, Michelle has been a great joy to our family. She is bright, funny, and sensitive. She won the "giggler's award" at a summer vacation program when she was four. She always sees the humor in everything. She is also very wise. I remember when she was six and we were driving past a house, she asked me, "Mommy, when you look at that house you see a blue house, and when I look at that house I see a blue house, but how do I know that we are seeing the same thing?" Although she is an honor student at the University of Chicago and has read and mastered all the primary sources that she had to read for her courses, her favorite books are still Antoine de Saint-Exupery's *The Little Prince* and Benjamin Hoff's *The Tao of Pooh*.

Michelle has always been very artistic and did calligraphy very well. She would copy sayings that expressed her philosophy of life and hang them around her room or paste them on the back of her door. One of her favorites was, "Die when I may, I want it to be said of me by those who knew me best, that I always plucked a thistle and planted a flower where I thought a flower would grow." This quote gets to the core of her very being. I've always thought of Michelle as a flower child, not in the sixties sense, but in the way that she always seems to brighten up the space and the people around her. She truly loves life and everything about it. But now perhaps at only twenty-one she might lose her life. I knew that there was a good chance that she might already be dead even as we sat on this plane waiting to reach her. And so I started to plan her funeral and searched through my training attempting to find concepts that might help me deal with her death. My head has always led my heart especially when I have limited amounts of energy. The emotional components get put on hold. Now as I sat on the plane I found myself resorting to my familiar pattern.

It was ironic. All week, I had been working on a book proposal with a working title of "Loosening the Ties that Bind: Towards a Theology of Children." As a mother who had gone back to graduate school late in life, I discovered how little the field of theology had reflected on the work of parenting. Yet I knew firsthand what important moral activity parenting was. Recently, however, some very important scholarly work was beginning to appear on family issues and the moral endeavor of parenting. I wanted to contribute to this field.

In all the theological literature, authors always said that children were gifts, not possessions, and that as parents we were only their stewards, not their owners. As parents, we have ties that bind us to our children, but these ties can be neither too loose, for this leads to neglecting our children, nor too tight. Although there has been much written about how we as a society are neglecting our children and all the problems that result from this, little has been written about what it means to hold on to our children too tightly. This was where I intended to focus my work, because my youngest child was old enough and mature enough to be on her own, and I knew how difficult it was for me to let her go. I never suspected, however, that the letting go might be a final gesture. But now it was time to reflect on that. What did it mean to believe that a child is a gift?

The first question that came to mind was a gift from whom? If someone or something is a gift there needs to be a gift giver. As a theologian it was easy for me to answer this question because theology teaches that all that is comes from God. Everything that we have has been freely given to us by God, and we are not entitled to any of it but are to receive it gratefully. The mystery of course is why some individuals who desperately want a child and work very hard to conceive discover that they cannot while others who did not intend to bring forth new life find themselves pregnant. We need to remember, however, that the one who gives cannot be controlled by the desire of the receiver. One does not have to give just because someone wants to receive. Gifts are freely given and the decision to give lies solely with the giver. This is what makes it a gift. It is not owed to us. Recognizing a child as gift draws us into the mystery and wonderment of creation and pushes us beyond the boundaries of justice.

I realized that not everyone would agree with this. There are many reasons people have children and many different values that societies put on children. In some cultures, especially in agrarian societies, children are viewed as economic assets. In our culture, children are often prized for their emotional value. Parents often look to their children as a source of satisfaction and of pride. How often do we hear parents say, "My son, the doctor," "My daughter, the lawyer," or view the rear windows of cars plastered with decals from prestigious universities, or bumper stickers that remind us that their children are on honor rolls. Other parents view children as burdens who interfere with their lifestyle. There is even the case of the father who impregnated his wife specifically to later kill the child in order to wreak revenge on his wife. These different views of children would lead to different reactions should one's child be in danger of dying or becoming severely brain damaged.

It was because I had been taught that children are gifts and because I truly accepted this concept that my reaction was as it was. The fact that I viewed Michelle as a gift and I viewed my family and community as having been gifted by Michelle led me to respond the way I did throughout this ordeal. I realized that Michelle had been given to me by another and that she was in my care only–not in my possession. But this led me to my next question. What did it mean to receive a gift? There is always the possibility of refusing a gift. But we had not. We had graciously welcomed Michelle into our lives and with that came the responsibility to care for her. She was a gift that could not be put on a shelf and admired or in a drawer and ignored but a gift that reminded us every day that by accepting her we entered into a relationship of caring. She was not ours to do with as we wished but she was entrusted to our care by another. Bonds were formed around her – bonds to the one who gave her to us, bonds to her, and bonds to all of those who were part of her life. We were all in this plane rushing to be with her because of those bonds and the love that they ignited. She was our daughter and our sister. I thought of the words in *The Little Prince*: " It is the time you have wasted on your rose that makes your rose so important." It was the time that we had all spent together and the bonds that we had formed that made us so special to each other. That's what makes the concept of gift so important.

Not only does accepting the gift of another connect you to the giver but it means opening yourself to the hurts, the joys, everything about the other. I realized that at this point there was little we could do to help Michelle. She was in the hands of skilled physicians yet we all knew we needed to be there, to be present as much for us as for her. And although we were the ones on the plane rushing to be with her it was obvious that she was not just a gift to us but to an entire community. A community had embraced her and was now drawn into this adventure as well. As the story unfolded, I would come more and more to realize how important this community would be not only to her but to all of us. Recognizing Michelle as a gift in our lives and coming to some deeper understanding as to what that meant laid the framework for everything that was to follow.

As we approached Chicago, a calmness enveloped me as I thought about Michelle as a gift and me as her caretaker. This helped me come to terms with the fact that she might be dead when we arrived at the hospital, and that I would need to let her go. But I was no longer frightened. I realized that I was not in control of this dramatic event, and that this was part of something much bigger than Michelle, my family, or me. We were only the actors, and the playwright had not informed us of the developing plot or of the play's end. We had to give the performance of our lives without any assurance as to where our roles would take us. We had to trust, to give ourselves over to the direction of another, to believe that, no matter what happened, someone was in charge and would only do what was best for us. And we needed to do all this without a script.

As I departed the plane I realized that there was only one promise that I could make to my daughter. That was: "No matter what happens Michelle you will never go through this alone. I will always be with you for you are my daughter and I am your mother."

2.

The Arrival

The flight was uneventful. We arrived at O'Hare Airport in Chicago sometime between 10 and 11 pm. We had not checked any luggage so we were able to depart rapidly. The airport was nearly deserted when we arrived, and I ran to a phone to try to reach our oldest son, Nick. Someone had already told him about the accident, and he had booked a 6 am flight to Chicago. After speaking with Nick, I just wanted to rush to the hospital, but Larry was intent on calling our answering service and checking messages. He listened to every message that had arrived since our departure. I wondered if he was trying to find out if Michelle was already dead so he could prepare himself during the drive to the hospital. Finally, we all hopped into a cab and told the driver to take us to Cook County Hospital.

When we arrived at the hospital, I could not believe what I saw. The hospital was old, decrepit, dirty, in a bad part of the city, and we had to climb over homeless people and drug addicts to get through the lobby. I kept saying,

"Why here? Why did they bring Michelle here?" I found out later that Cook County was the nearest trauma 1 hospital. Even though Michelle's accident happened only a few blocks from the University of Chicago Hospital, it had no trauma room. Cook County is famous for its trauma room, although I didn't know that at the time.

As we walked into the lobby, I saw a group of Michelle's friends huddled off to the side. They all looked relieved that we had arrived. I asked if anyone else had been hurt, and they told me four other students had been hit as well. Three had been released from the hospital, and the fourth was at Northwestern University Hospital, but they didn't know how he was. They then took me to a back room where I saw more of Michelle's friends and her resident head, Paul. They told us that the surgery was over, and Michelle was still alive. Then they took us to Michelle's doctor, Margaret McGregor, who told us that the surgeons had removed a hematoma from the right side of Michelle's brain and that they were keeping a close watch on the other side of her brain for another possible dangerous hematoma. My health-care training kicked in, and the first question I asked was whether there had ever been a lack of oxygen to her brain. I was told that she was still breathing on her own when the ambulance arrived and was intubated on the way to the hospital. Michelle had arrived at the hospital a three on the Glasgow Coma Scale, which is the lowest you can be without being declared brain dead. Dr. McGregor also informed us that the next forty-eight hours were crucial as to whether Michelle would live or die.

With that short introduction, we followed Dr. McGregor to the neuro ICU unit on the third floor. On the way, I told the doctor that I teach health-care ethics. I don't know why I said that. I was thinking aloud and attempting to organize what my family was experiencing by trying to fit this extraordinary event into neat ethical categories. I was searching for any method I could find to bring some kind of order to what was occurring. I knew about these situations. I use case studies in my classroom and had taught about Karen Ann Quinlan and Nancy Beth Cruzan, both young women who were unconscious for long periods of time and then eventually died when treatment was withdrawn. In the back of my mind there was a fleeting thought that this could possibly be our fate. I pondered how to bring what I know professionally to bear on my family's situation. How do I fit my professional and personal worlds together? Is this what my training had prepared me for or would it be better to know less?

As we entered the neuro ICU unit, I saw one large room filled with about ten beds and its occupants. Next to one sat a policeman, guarding a sleeping man. In another was a man with a halo screwed into his head. Many people were connected to respirators and there were beeps and noises that I had never heard before. In the corner next to a window was Michelle, or so they told me. It was hard to recognize her. She was lying in a bed with a respirator in her mouth. Her head was covered with white bandages and a tube protruded from the middle of her skull. It was attached to a machine that measured her intercranial pressure. Her right eye was swollen and it looked like part of her brain had been pushed forward behind her right eye. There were tubes attached to every part of her body. In fact, the only parts of her body that I could touch were the toes on her right foot.

I looked at my sons and husband. They were close to tears. The reflection I had done on the plane helped me, and as I walked over and hugged each of them

I told them that, no matter what happened, we had had a beautiful gift for twenty-one years, and no one could ever take that from us.

After some time, my husband and the boys left to find us a place to stay for the night. But I was fixated on the bed, my daughter, the nurse who cared for her, and the machines. Every time something beeped, I jumped but I was constantly reassured as the nurse who cared for Michelle calmly went and readjusted something, took down notes, and kept a close eye on the numbers on her machines. Her calmness reassured me, and I will never forget her. I don't think she once left my daughter's bedside all night. I sat on a chair at the bottom of the bed and spent the night kissing Michelle's toes, frightened that at any moment the beeps would stop and Michelle would be dead.

Around three o'clock in the morning, I thought of my mother. If Michelle should die, the first question my mother would ask me was whether she had received the sacrament of the sick, or, as my mother would refer to it, the last rites. I had not even thought of that before, but now it haunted me. I asked the nurse whether there was a Catholic chaplain on duty. I was told that he could not be reached until 7 am. I asked her whether she thought we could wait until then to get him, but she was not sure. I went into the waiting room and found several of Michelle's friends and her resident head still there. I told them of my dilemma, and one of them called his parish priest who came to the hospital in the middle of the night and anointed my daughter.

Thinking of my mother also made me intent on contacting the woman who hit Michelle. I had found out that she was an elderly woman who had lost control of her car. She had side-swiped three students at the bottom of the hill in front of Michelle's dorm and then panicked, soaring her car up the hill where she caught Michelle's leg under her front tire, dragging Michelle about forty feet, and plowing her car into a wall while hitting another student who went through her front windshield. I knew if the driver had been my mother, she could never live with herself, and I wanted this driver to know that I understood that this was an accident, albeit a terrible one.

No one searches for tragedy, but as I sat at the bottom of Michelle's bed I felt myself pushed out of the daily routine of ordinary existence. Before we received the phone call tonight I had so much to do. I make lists and cross things off as I do them. The list I had made for the upcoming week was exceptionally long. When the phone call arrived, however, I forgot the list, got on a plane, and had no idea when I would be returning to New York. But it didn't matter. Nothing on that list, which seemed so important only a short time ago mattered anymore. All that mattered now was the moment and being at my daughter's bedside. As I listened to the beeps and alarms, time stood still. I was totally focused on my daughter and trying to let her know that I was there.

Michelle survived the night, and in the morning I met her attending physicians, Dr. Glick and Dr. Stone. They advised us of the seriousness of Michelle's condition, but there was little we could do but stand by and wait. As the morning progressed I was pulled back into the daily routine and again reminded that there were things I needed to take care of. I knew there were people at home wondering how things were progressing.

The only phones to which I had access were pay phones in the corridor around the corner from the ICU. I had a calling card and began what would turn into a daily routine of notifying friends and relatives of what was going on. I called Father Ruiz at St. John's and let him know of the seriousness of the accident. I called Aunt Noreen and my sister. Nick arrived from New York and saw his sister for the first time. Larry and the other two boys came, and around 11 am I went to the hotel room, which was about two blocks away, and tried to get some sleep, but it was impossible. My mind was racing, and about 2 pm I returned to the hospital.

When I returned I found the waiting room teeming with people from the university: officials, teachers, friends and acquaintances. Everyone was coming to realize the seriousness of the accident and wanted to be at the hospital. They indicated to me how loved and admired Michelle was. I heard stories of what she had done as an RA (resident assistant) from baking bread every day in the bread machine in her room to listening for hours to the problems and concerns of those on her floor. Her friends told me of the fun they had always had together and I thought of the saying posted on her wall: "He who laughs, lasts."

Professors informed me of the excellence of her work and one gave me a term paper she had written on the mind-body dualism and individuality as addressed by John Dewey. Her paper was prescient of what we were experiencing. In her paper, Michelle highlighted Dewey's objection to egotism – the belief in an isolated ego belonging to an individual body, which leads to selfishness, discontent with surroundings, and a resulting turn to the "inner world". She then writes about a personal experience. In her words: "My personal experience with psychological counseling offers an especially illustrative example. During my second year of college, a very close friend admitted to me that she was extremely depressed. After talking to her about it and trying to help, I felt

drained and wanted some guidance on the most effec-
tive way to aid her. I went to see a counselor here at the
university, and when I told her I was there for advice on
helping a depressed friend one of her first questions was,
'Why do you feel like you have to help your friend?' I had
no answer for her; I was not expecting that question at
all. As the session went on, this stress on the isolated ego
and turning inward became apparent. I was being treated
like an individual independent of my surroundings and it
became clear that I was not expected to be able to help
my friend very much because she was another isolated
ego that had to turn inward in order to overcome depression." She continues, "Most of today's clinical psychology
calls for a divorce from environment, where Dewy calls
for continuity, connection, and wholeness. I cannot
help but wonder how this philosophy could change the
face of psychology." I felt like we were about to find out
because it was connection to others that was giving us
the strength to go through this ordeal and I suspected
Michelle's survival hinged on her continued connection
to us. She stated in her paper, "Mind resides in interaction and activity, not inside an organism but around it." If
that is the case then we have an important role to play in
keeping her engaged.

The conclusion of her paper also gave me hope to face
the day. She wrote: "This paper represents, as Dewey might
say, an end. In a sense it marks the conclusion of an activity, namely attending this class and working on this specific material. But the end of one activity can always be the
beginning of something else, something more; ends 'are
employed to give activity added meaning and to direct its
further course…they are redirecting pivots in action' (HNC
155). So *an* end is not *the* end but a beginning too, a small
mark in the continuous process of learning."

As I reflected on her paper, Michelle continued to sleep in the ICU. We continued to wait out the forty-eight hours, and I spent Monday night trying to sleep in the waiting room. In the waiting room there were seats connected by metal bars, a vending machine, and an old TV bolted to a corner wall. It was impossible to get comfortable in these chairs, which were dirty and stained. A steady stream of patients kept entering the room during the night to get snacks from the vending machine. In the room with me were family members of other patients. The doctor on call slept in a little room next to our waiting room, and any time he or she was called to the ICU unit, we would all jump and run in to see whose family member was in crisis.

Tuesday morning a reporter from *Newsday*, our Long Island newspaper, called about Michelle. We had a friend who worked for *Newsday* and I assumed that Bob was the one who notified the paper of Michelle's accident. The eventual article was titled, "A Moment of Grace." For me, grace is experiencing the presence of God and even though we were going through a life-changing event its tragic weight was lightened by the presence and support of others. God came to me through others and I can't remember any time in my life when my family and I had felt more loved.

Later in the day, Michelle underwent another CAT (computed tomography) scan. The doctor informed me of the results and then left the room. The scan showed that the hematoma on the left side of Michelle's brain seemed to resolve itself. Within minutes of giving me that information, the doctor rushed back in with a consent form for me to sign for Michelle's surgery. Michelle's brain had begun to swell, and the doctors were able to reduce it temporarily with medication, but they had a small window of time in which to do surgery. I'll never forget the consent form: next to "possible side effects," was "death"; next to "alternatives," was "none." I signed. The team began running down the corridor with a nurse next to Michelle, manually working a respirator while another nurse yelled, "clear the way, clear the way." All I could do was sit down and wait. I was so numb I couldn't even pray. I went to the pay phone in the hall, and I called a friend in New York to ask her how she had gotten through a similar ordeal. My friend's son had been injured as a young child and was unconscious for a time. There was no answer, but I left a message on my friend's answering machine.

Here I was signing consent forms for my daughter and I realized the cool, methodical way I had presented these forms in the classroom bore little resemblance to what it is actually like to sign these forms. Much of my ethical training in health care had focused on the principle of autonomy. This principle states that individuals should have the right to make their own decisions. All kinds of instruments such as health-care proxies, living wills, durable powers of attorney, etc. are put in place to guarantee that even when someone becomes unconscious his or her wishes will be carried out. But Michelle had none of these documents, as most twenty-one year olds don't think of dying. I needed to give my consent, as her surrogate, based on what I thought was best for Michelle and what I thought she would have wanted. I was now faced with the reality of signing consent forms for Michelle's procedures even though I knew that I was not giving informed consent. Informed consent means that one has sufficient information, comprehends the information, and is not coerced into making the decision. There also needs to be a sufficient amount of time to reflect on this information.

When Michelle arrived at the hospital, the doctors made the decision to operate on her, a decision I learned later could have gone either way. Because she was so close to death and so badly injured when she arrived at the hospital, some had thought that surgery might be futile. Others questioned the quality of life that would result from surgery. Yes, the physicians called our family in New York before they operated, but the decision had already been made to rush Michelle into surgery and how could we possibly ascertain in New York whether that was the appropriate decision. Even if we had been in Chicago, at this phase we were totally dependent on the physicians' decisions.

Likewise, even now that we were at Cook County Hospital, I simply signed the forms the doctors gave me. I had no idea what any of it meant or how to make an informed decision regarding the procedures. When I was told that Michelle would die if she did not have surgery immediately, how could I not sign? The physicians too, I suspect, were only reacting to what needed to be done in the moment to save her life. The fallout would come later. What discussions they had among themselves I do not know. I went along with their recommendations because I had no choice. Yes, I understood informed consent. Yes, the appropriate forms were given to me (although I did not see anyone else sign consent forms). No, I didn't give informed consent, but we all pretended that I did. Signing consent forms was an illusionary symbol that we had control over the situation, but we were all taking our cues from Michelle and only reacting to what needed to be done. I learned from this that the overriding ethical question is not who should be the one to decide what should be done but rather how can we all, professionals and family, rise to the occasion. Even though Michelle was unconscious, she and her needs were the center of everything. She was the one who gave the rest of us purpose. While Michelle was in the operating room, I again found myself reflecting on my professional knowledge and testing how it matched my experience.

Michelle returned from the operating room, and a new forty-eight-hour waiting period started. The waiting room was again packed with University of Chicago students and personnel. In addition, phone calls kept going back and forth between New York and Chicago. It was hard for anyone to reach me, although the switchboard did let several calls come through to the ICU unit. I made most of the calls from the pay phones in the hall. The fact that Michelle's primary care physician was also a friend eased things for us because he had immediate access to her condition.

Our son Tim returned home on Tuesday to take care of details such as bill paying and cash access and availability. The family in New York was also dealing with my father-in-law, who was still unconscious in Glen Cove Community Hospital ICU. I again spent Tuesday night in the waiting room with family members of other patients.

Wednesday was somewhat quiet. Michelle was stable although still unconscious. I continued to sleep in the waiting room, talk to the physicians during the day, greet the visitors who came, and spend much time next to my daughter's bed. In addition, some of Michelle's friends from Long Island began to arrive. What a boost it was to come out of the ICU and find a new arrival. Just as I would begin to doubt or feel hopeless someone new would arrive and recharge me. I learned too that the people of our community were keeping a constant prayer vigil at our church, St. Boniface Martyr in Sea Cliff. Someone was there around the clock praying for Michelle and us. While I was sitting with Michelle, someone was sitting with me many miles away.

On Thursday, the doctors informed me that they were still not happy with the swelling on Michelle's brain, and they told me they were going to put her into a barbiturate coma to lower the swelling. This was extremely dangerous because it would again bring Michelle close to death, but there seemed to be no alternative. An EEG machine was attached to Michelle to keep track of her brain waves.

On Thursday evening, I was sitting by Michelle's bedside when a phone call from our son Tim came through to the ICU unit. He informed me that my father-in-law had died. Truthfully, thoughts of my father-in-law had left my mind as I focused on my daughter but I recognized how difficult this would be for my husband. I called the hotel and asked my sons and husband to come to the hospital. I was careful to begin by saying it's not Michelle. Again, I did not want to tell them this news over the phone. When they arrived, we went to a little snack area and I informed them that Papa had died. My poor husband – his father had just died in New York – his daughter was dying in Chicago—and there was also the family business to consider. We tried to think of what we would do, but we were too overwhelmed and put off all decisions until the next day. The men went back to the hotel, and I went back to my daughter's bedside. I sat down and wrote a letter to my colleagues at St. John's. My friend Rose made a copy of it and saved it for me. After describing the events of the previous days, and informing them of my father-in-law's death, this is what I wrote:

Sitting, sleeping, spending most of my days in the neuro waiting room, I'm rubbing elbows with all kinds of people. There's the family of the young man who was shot in the head while stopped at a traffic light. He's been shot three times before. He survived. His father, Tommy, told me where to buy the best "soul food" in Chicago. Then there's Dorothy who arrives every morning by bus at 5am to be with her daughter who's recovering from a brain tumor. There's also the large Hispanic family who makes sure there is always a family member present, so when their 85-year-old father/grandfather comes out of his coma there will be someone there to help him and speak to him in Spanish. Mixed with these people you have the 15 to 20 students from the University of Chicago who spend time with us every day. There are always some of them who stay overnight. The students are teaching the families of the other groups about anatomy, anthropology, etc. They're also learning a good deal about the lives of these families. We're even watching Jerry Springer together.

It's amazing what is going on out here. I may not be with my St. John's students, but I'm spending my days and nights with these kids. Some have shaved their heads to be with Michelle. They've created Web pages, written songs, done art work, made cards, baked cookies, talked for hours with me, questioned the meaning of life. They've read to Michelle (everything from Winnie the Pooh to economics books), sung to her, recited poetry, acted out skits. We've developed our own little family in the waiting room. Even the hospital staff stops in to be with us because there is much laughter and little crying. They're practicing community, and I know that God is in our midst. We're our own little church.

I thank you all for your wonderful support with a special thanks to Dick, Jo Ann and Rose, who I understand, are teaching my classes. I don't know how everything *will turn out, but I do know this has been a moment of grace. Just as Hillary's in battle-mode in Washington, I'm in battle-mode in Chicago. We are fighting to save Michelle's life with every ounce of strength that we have — not because we can't let her go, but because the world would be a less beautiful place without her.*

Pray for us.

Marilyn

While I asked others to pray for us I found it difficult to pray myself. Although Larry found solace in going to the chapel on the sixth floor of the hospital, it was by sitting at my daughter's bedside and through others that God came to me. The Scriptural story that I clung to was the story of Jesus in the Garden of Gethsemane. Here we find our God preparing for the suffering that He knows lies ahead. He asks His disciples to pray with Him. When He finds them sleeping He is overcome with grief. He needed their companionship and their support. I found my light in my connectedness to my God's suffering and need for companionship.

The few times that I did pray I realized that my prayer had changed. For much of my life I had prayed to God to grant me what I wanted. Now, however, when the nurses told me to pray for a miracle, I got annoyed. That was an indication to me that there was little hope. I wanted good medical care from the medical staff, not encouragement to pray.

I also did not agree with the people who would say that I just needed to have faith and all would work out well. I didn't think that I had more faith than Mrs. Quinlan or Mrs. Cruzan and both of their daughters died. I refused to put myself into that bind. If I did and Michelle should die, it would mean that either I didn't have enough faith, or God could not prevent her death. Neither option was acceptable to me. This tragedy was so overwhelming that I was afraid to tell God what to do. Is it better that Michelle die or remain persistently vegetative? Is it better that she be vegetative or emerge severely brain injured? I was no longer even sure that a total cure was the answer for I came to appreciate that something worse might lie ahead for her. For the first time in my life Jesus' prayer became my prayer, "Thy will be done." It was not that I had become more spiritual but that I had become more aware of my limitations. I simply prayed that I would have the strength to face whatever might lie ahead for us. I also prayed that others would not desert me for what I did know beyond a shadow of a doubt was that it was other people's prayers that gave me the strength to go on. I needed to respond, not control. My worldview was shifting from doing to being. There was little I could do but wait and be present and I needed others to be present to me. As Pooh says in *The Tao of Pooh*: "Well we keep looking for Home and not finding it, so I thought that if we looked for this Pit, we'd be sure not to find it, which would be a Good Thing, because then we might find something that we weren't looking for, which might be just what we were looking for, really."

Michelle was the one who had brought hundreds of people together, both those of us who were present by her side and those who were with us in spirit. People who had not been in a church or who had not said a prayer in years were suddenly on their knees beseeching God for mercy. By lying in bed, unconscious to us all, she was calling forth the better parts of us that some of us had forgotten we had. Her grandfather would have been proud.

3.

Cook County Hospital

More of Michelle's friends from home began to arrive. Her childhood friend, Kara, had arrived from Geneseo University. Friday, Tamara came from Holy Cross College with her mother, Joan, Kristen came from Dayton University, and Mike flew in from Boston. Michelle's boyfriend's parents also came from Minnesota. Among the visitors that day was Sister Sheila Lyme, a Sister of Mercy based in Chicago, who had been contacted by the principal at Michelle's high school, Our Lady of Mercy Academy. (Michelle's friends had called the principal to inform her of the accident and Michelle's condition.) I found out later that Sister Sheila was also the Commissioner of Public Health for the City of Chicago.

Michelle was stable in her barbiturate coma, and we all sat in the waiting room, reminiscing about events in the past and waiting for news. Tamara and Kristin reminded us that the summer before they and Michelle had taken a tour of what they considered to be the stupidest places of their high school years. The evening ended when a policeman stopped them for going through a red light. They filmed the entire evening and promised to show us the film. It was during the same summer that Michelle gave a surprise twenty-first birthday party for Tamara at our house. I remembered that Michelle had arrived home at five-thirty and the party began at six.

On one of the cards that her friends made for her was a picture of Michelle dressed for a party as "medicine man," with white wrapping around her head, very similar to how she looked now. It was Michelle's sense of humor and her ability to see the light side of things that helped us now. In fact, her friends wanted to take pictures of her because they knew that should she wake up she would laugh at how she looked, wired and wrapped in the hospital bed.

Listening to them reminded me of how much Michelle always tried to pack into her days before the accident. She was always on the go. Everything about life interested her. In high school she was the editor of the school newspaper and involved in many extra curricular activities. During her summers she usually did some kind of volunteer work. She and Tamara spent two weeks one summer working in Williamsburg, Virginia, in a program called Landmark Volunteers. Michelle actually painted fences and laid brick in 100-degree weather. Another summer she worked at an International Peace Camp in Rhode Island. She brought three of the European volunteers home with her at the end of the stint so they would have a chance to see New York before they returned to Europe.

Another summer she worked at St. Christopher – Ottilie in Sea Cliff. This is a home that cares for children with disabilities. It was her work here that led her to minor in American Sign Language in college.

In college she was also very active. She edited the university's *Women's Guide to Health*, served as a class marshal, played intramural sports, and was an RA and consistent dean's list student. In addition, she volunteered in a local inner-city school. I remember the day she called me and told me that she had been demoted from first grade. Michelle had decided that the best way to deal with the disruptive children was to let them run around until they were tired and then they would sit down and complete their lesson. Needless to say, the principal thought otherwise, and told Michelle that perhaps she would be better working in kindergarten.

It was this love of life and her wonder at all different kinds of experiences and her appreciation of all different kinds of people that made us feel so comfortable at Cook County. Michelle truly understood diversity and saw goodness in everyone and everything. Another quote on her wall captured this: "How far you go in life depends on your being tender with the young, compassionate with the aged, sympathetic with the striving, and tolerant of the weak and strong because some day in life you will have been all of them."

As we reflected on these stories we also tried to plan how we would handle my father-in-law's funeral. Our son Larry decided to go home, and our son Nick would stay with me. My husband was still debating what to do.

Larry kept using the pay phone in the hall trying to get a flight home at a reduced rate. Because he had not asked for medical emergency rates when flying out, he was unable to get a reduced rate on the same airline to go home. He'd keep coming back to the waiting room to update us. Finally, he came back excited. He had found a reduced rate. We asked how. "Bereavement," he replied. Our black humor kicked in. Ah, bereavement. So much had happened during the week that we had forgotten that we had more than one reason for emergency airline rates.

On Saturday, our son Larry flew home, and my husband decided that he would leave the following day so that he could be present at his father's wake on Sunday evening and attend the funeral on Monday. Nick and I would take care of things in Chicago. My husband wanted to be there for his father but I think he was afraid of breaking down when people approached him at the wake. So he went at the end when only the immediate family was there. He was also aware that his daughter might die while he was in New York.

I found more irony in our situation. My entire life I had prayed for the strength to be a helpmate to my husband when his father died. Papa had a very strong personality and I knew his death would leave a large gap in the family. In addition, my husband was the oldest of the next generation so everyone would look to him to take charge, especially in the business. Now I was not even there with him. He had to go through this without me.

Visitors kept coming and going all weekend, and Michelle continued to sleep peacefully in her barbiturate coma. On Sunday, the out-of-towners left, and my husband went home to New York, but we were still surrounded by many faithful friends from the University of Chicago. The students had begun a sign-in book and wrote notes to Michelle whenever they came to visit. By now, the walls of the waiting room were covered with posters and get-well cards. Some friends had even rented time in a recording studio and made a tape of original songs for Michelle. Michelle and her story were becoming quite well known throughout the hospital.

Cook County was a hospital like no other I had seen. Here the guards carried guns, the patients walked through the halls and the lobby in their hospital gowns dragging their IV poles. There was no cafeteria, only vending machines with a Starbucks coffee bar in the lobby. Other than the ICU and specialized rooms, there were no private rooms, and no air conditioning. Often the elevators didn't work and the floors were dirty. Yet this is the hospital that had the nation's first blood bank, has one of the finest burn centers, and a large neo-natal intensive-care unit, and what we were especially grateful for, a world-class trauma center. I read about 5,000 patients came through the trauma room every year. It sees many who have gunshot wounds because of the hospital's location near neighborhoods heavily controlled by gangs. This is the hospital that the television show "ER" was based on. Cook County truly is a legend.

On the third floor where we were there were only two toilets that we all used, the patients, the outpatients who came for therapy, and those of us in the waiting room. They were dirty, the toilet seat was broken on one of them, and the door did not close all the way but I used it. That was something I would worry about later.

So many people who talked to me in the waiting room told me how very grateful they were for Cook County Hospital. Although to an outsider it appeared as a rundown, dilapidated old building, in fact it is sometimes referred to as "The Old Lady of Harrison Street," to those who sought care there, it was their source of hope. When one had nowhere else to go, Cook County opened its doors.

Yet it certainly had a roughness to it that was also a reflection of the population it served. Multiple victims of shootings are not what I have ever seen at a hospital.

Added to that, though less dramatic, a gang member marked Michelle's sign-in book, someone stole her tape recorder, and Jerry Springer was the favorite television program, with the young women in the waiting room yelling "You go girl," when fights broke out on the show. I had experienced enough of that aspect of the hospital to retain a realistic view of it and the people who sought care there.

On Monday morning, Dr. Glick informed me that they had taken Michelle out of her barbiturate coma and all we could do was wait for her to wake up. I called home, and my son Tim relayed the message to the family members who were all gathered for lunch after my father-in-law's funeral. We had buried one member of the family, but because Michelle seemed to be on the road to recovery, we had cause for joy. Things were looking up. We would wait for Michelle to awaken and then send her to rehabilitation. Hopefully things would be back to normal soon.

Dr. Glick also informed me that I could transfer Michelle to another hospital if I wished. Although I had been talking to doctors from the University of Chicago Hospital, I decided to keep Michelle at Cook County as long as she was in the ICU unit, where she would receive good care. I felt that these surgeons had saved Michelle's life, and I also knew that we were one of the few families in the hospital who had insurance. I hoped to bring scarce resources to the hospital. Perhaps I made this decision because I teach in a university run by the Vincentian Order, whose mission is to serve the poor. I decided we would continue this journey surrounded by the poor. Besides at this point I thought it wouldn't be long before Michelle would awaken and we would be leaving.

All that week, I continued my watch by Michelle's bedside, but there was no evidence that she was emerging from the coma. The only change in our routine was that I began to go to the hotel around 10 pm until 6 am to sleep while my son Nick stayed by Michelle's bedside. I also was getting to know many more individuals at Cook County. What I noticed was that most of the individuals in the waiting room, both those who were there for long periods of time and those who only stayed a short time, had a deep, spiritual faith - a belief that no matter what happened they were not alone, but God was with them. They prayed openly, they expressed their faith and hope to each other constantly. They supported each other, and even though their children were called "fast mama" or "big girl," they got up early in the morning and spent hours on public transportation to be with them. Gang members had large extended families that cared about them, and when someone died, they cried, they prayed, they moved on. Life was hard, but life also held value and joy. They seldom complained but rather constantly praised God.

Our cousin Mary Ann visited on Wednesday of that week. She was on her way back to California from my father-in-law's funeral. Mary Ann is a neurobiologist who does post-doctoral work in the neurosciences. She was able to examine Michelle's CAT scans and get a detailed explanation from Michelle's doctor as to her condition. Supposedly there was nothing on her scans to indicate that she would not awaken although we did know that there was a great deal of brain damage.

We waited and waited. The doctors told us to begin to look for rehabilitation facilities, and I knew that I wanted Michelle to go to the Rehabilitation Institute of Chicago (RIC). It was one of the best in the country, and we were already in Chicago. But I didn't understand anything about rehabilitation. I had always thought rehab was for drug or alcohol abuse. In addition, people began to use terms like acute, sub-acute, skilled nursing. I knew nothing about these distinctions. All I knew was that somehow Michelle was going to RIC. I wouldn't even consider another facility. My daughter was going to go to the best.

But here again was a professional/personal conflict. I believed wholeheartedly in social justice and an equitable distribution of health care yet as I was planning to fight for Michelle's admittance to RIC I realized no one else in the ICU would ever be able to go there. County patients went to county facilities for rehab.

Here at Cook County, Michelle's physical condition was a great leveler of economic status. As she lay dying, material possessions were unimportant. The surgeons did the same surgery on my daughter as they did on the gang member who arrived with three tears tattooed under his eye (each tear signifying someone he had killed). But when it came time to be discharged, money mattered tremendously. The system is run by insurance, and without it you cannot receive services. No matter how compassionate individual health-care workers might be, they have little ability to change the system. You lose your individuality and become a cog in the wheel that is fueled by your insurance coverage. I knew that RIC would not accept anyone without health insurance.

Before I could reflect on this more, the doctors informed me that they had hoped the fluid on Michelle's brain would dissipate but it had not, so they needed to place a shunt in her head. This shunt would drain the fluid off of her brain into a medical bag by her bedside. This was another setback but we were hopeful that this would be only a temporary measure. Michelle looked peaceful and calm lying in her bed. The swelling of her eye had receded, and the white wraps had been removed from her head, which was completely shaved. If there is a positive side to brain injury it is that you are not watching your loved one suffer. Throughout the constant turmoil at Cook County, Michelle always looked very angelic. She slept peacefully through everything. I thought of the quote from *The Little Prince*, "it is only with the heart that one can see rightly; what is essential is invisible to the eye."

But the turmoil continued around her. During this time, there was much happening in the waiting room. During the day, cancer patients would come for chemotherapy, and AIDS patients would come for treatment. They would line up in the hall and the overflow or those who were too ill to stand would come into the waiting room. Because of the posters on the walls and the presence of our family and friends, they came to know Michelle, and we came to know some of their stories. I'll never forget the single mother who came for chemo after she had sent her daughter to school and then went to her job as a waitress after treatment. She could barely stand and yet needed to go to work to support herself and her daughter.

There was also a young man who kept coming in for shunt adjustments, and I kept wondering whether this was the future that Michelle would have in store. But I couldn't think of the future; I could only get through the day. I remember yelling at Dr. Stone when he pointed out all the complications that could lie ahead for Michelle. I told him that he knew all the possibilities, but they were only that – possibilities.

I began to see some very subtle changes among those around us. After Michelle's boyfriend's parents visited I noticed him begin to pull back from his visits to

Michelle. I suspected that his parents had come down to assess the situation and had advised their son to begin to distance himself from Michelle. Was she now considered damaged goods? I understood their concerns but I resented it. What happened to Michelle could happen to anyone. What if we all began to walk away from those who needed our help? I also observed how frequently people would tell me that I needed to take care of myself. They were not volunteering to sit by Michelle's bedside so I could get some rest, they were advising me to walk away, to begin distancing myself. The day the hospital psychologist came to me and told me that perhaps I should go out to the museum for the afternoon I blew up at him. I informed him that I was very capable of knowing what I needed and when I had some needs he could help me with I would let him know. How do I walk around a museum when my daughter might die while I am there?

Are we so indoctrinated by Darwin's premise of "the survival of the fittest" that once we judge someone may require care from us or put excessive demands on us, we begin to withdraw? I thought about what makes us fit. It is often assumed that it is our genes. Isn't this what the eugenics movement was all about? Yet the more I thought about it I recognized that it is not just our genes but is directly related to who gets the best care. Care giving is so undervalued in our society that it often makes one appear less of a person if one needs care. From an early age we are taught to be self-sufficient and independent. Likewise because care-giving activity is either paid at a low wage or not at all, those who do this work also become vulnerable in society. Yet perhaps it was those species that were best at care giving that survived and developed. The higher one is in the order of primates the longer the period of care one needs to mature. I recognized that my promise to Michelle that she would not go through this alone might require a great deal of care giving on my part. Again I wondered if I was up to it.

That week we had a blizzard and I could barely walk to the hospital. The snow was coming down so strongly and with the winds, it hit you horizontally. When I walked into the hospital, the lights were flickering. I prayed the hospital's generator worked. My daughter was on a ventilator.

Our cousin Laurie arrived that week, and she went to work finding us a place to stay when Michelle was admitted to RIC. Laurie is like her mother, very methodical. She went to RIC and got a list of places to stay that were close by. I needed a place within close walking distance because I did not want to take a taxi every day. Both of my knees needed replacement, and I was in excruciating pain whenever I walked. I would often have to stop and rest in the middle of walking the two blocks to the hospital. Laurie came back with a list of available places. She had also visited them all and listed the advantages and disadvantages of each. She recommended staying at the Sommerfield Suites, which was only two blocks from RIC and right next to Northwestern University Hospital. I would have a little kitchen, a bedroom, bath, and a living room with a pullout couch. This way when friends or relatives came there would also be a place for them to stay.

Things began to look promising again. Michelle seemed to be moving more, we had contacted RIC to begin the initial evaluation of Michelle for acceptance into their program, and I had found a place to stay.

And then it happened. The doctors informed me that Michelle's shunt had gotten infected and that they needed to rush her into surgery. I didn't exactly understand the seriousness of this at the time, but I later learned that it meant a serious infection had gotten into her brain and could kill her. I also learned that should she survive this surgery, she would probably need a permanent shunt. This would drain the fluid off of her brain into her stomach to prevent her from developing hydrocephalous. And then I knew that even if Michelle should live, our lives would never be the same. Her friends were beginning to go back to their normal routines (they were studying for finals), but we were facing quite a different future. There was a separation beginning to occur that felt like "us and them". It was as if we were being separated from life as we had known it. We were being pulled into another realm of reality.

Yet strangely, I never asked why this was happening to us. I knew that we were human and these things happen to humans no matter how much we try to pretend that they don't. Life is not all fun and games – it has some real challenges mixed in. What was most important to me was that we not go through this ordeal alone. I was overwhelmed by a need for community, and I found great consolation in hearing from others, whether through phone calls, which were difficult to receive, or the mail. It was equally important to me that I respond to people who contacted me. Writing letters, talking, reflecting, and staying in contact with others was what held me together. Many times, people would say to me that I should let them know if they said anything to me that upset me. What was important to me was that they were there, not what they said. I'm sure I said some rather strange things, because when you are experiencing this level of tragedy you do not censor your speech. You do not attempt to be politically correct, and who you are at your core comes through. All pretenses are gone, and you relate on a purely human level. When I responded to a letter from my dean, he was no longer Father O'Connell but Dave.

I called and contacted whomever I needed or felt a desire to talk to. At one point I remembered something Carolyn McCarthy had said after her husband was killed and her son was severely injured in the Long Island Railroad attack, and even though she had since become a congresswoman on Long Island, I wrote to her. I related to her as a mother and decided to reach out to her, just as I had called my friend Marianne because she had experienced a similar tragedy with her son. I had an overwhelming need to stay connected.

Laurie left to go home that day, but our Aunt Louise was coming out the following day. Aunt Louise brightens every place that she goes. She arrived with her cookies for the nurses, her Italian songs, and her general good cheer. She snuck a prime rib dinner from the hotel into the hospital for me, and made me eat it behind the pillar in the little vending room so no one would get jealous.

Michelle had survived the surgery but was still unconscious. Aunt Louise and I stood by her bedside, singing to her, reading to her, holding her hand, telling her how much we loved her.

Visitors continued to write in Michelle's sign-in-book. At first, they would sign only their names, but soon others – Michelle's friends as well as strangers – began to write messages. On March 13th I found the following message:

"Michelle I believe God's going to do a miracle in your life. Jesus loves you and he gives you life. I believe He's going to make you understand the precious gift of life. Consider my words and dedicate your life to Him. And He will bless you and use your testimony so many people will understand how beautiful is life. God is life. Carmelo, Puerto Rico."

The faith of the people surrounding me was palpable. Families here openly talked of their faith and raised their loved ones up in prayer. Families of gang members would gather in circles and pray for their loved one who had been shot in the head. And because I was in need, they had adopted me. The Hispanic woman who scrubbed the floors would bring me a carafe of coffee from her home every morning. The woman who operated the elevator often brought fried chicken that she had made for me. I came to realize the richness of these people's lives and knew that I would never call them poor again – perhaps economically poor – but certainly not poor in a spiritual sense.

I listened to people in the waiting room, and I learned that some of their problems consisted of not being able to afford some of the little things in life. For instance, Maria had learned that her husband was going to be discharged from the hospital but would need to come back for follow-up visits. On learning this news, she began to cry. She had not cried while he was undergoing treatment, but now the thought of getting him back to the hospital for scheduled treatment overwhelmed her. She could not afford a taxi, and he would be too weak to travel on a bus. How was she going to do this?

Many family friends and relatives with some economic means asked me what they could do for me. After listening to the people in the waiting room at the hospital, the idea came to me of setting up a fund in Michelle's name at Cook County that would be available to provide petty cash for things like transportation for patients who needed to return to the hospital for treatment. I knew we could not afford a wing of the hospital, but we could help in a little way. As I thought about this idea, I also knew that Michelle would want it to focus on children because she loved children. I spoke with Father John, the chaplain of the hospital, and he set up a meeting with a pediatrician in the hospital, and we opened the Michelle Martone Oncology Fund. We notified our friends in New York and Chicago and over time raised $10,000 for the children and their families at Cook County.

The wait for Michelle to wake up continued. And then on Saturday morning, March 14th, Michelle squeezed Aunt Louise's hand and mine when we asked her to. She was coming out. We both felt her squeeze. Aunt Louise was going home that day. What a wonderful farewell present. My friend Genie flew in that afternoon and would spend the weekend with me. Genie would be with me when Michelle woke up but soon after Genie's arrival Michelle began to shiver. We knew the fever was returning and the nurses put Michelle under an ice blanket. We could only hope. As soon as Michelle seemed to make some progress something else happened. There were times I was hungry for information and other times when I didn't want to know. This fit into the latter.

On Sunday, Dr. Glick stopped by in the early evening and did not like what she saw. She told me she was going to take Michelle back for more surgery. Evidently, Michelle had developed another shunt infection. I signed the consent form; Michelle was rushed to the operating room, and I lay down on the chairs. This was when I realized what a toll signing consent forms was taking on me. I did not have the energy to call my husband in New York, and Genie had to do it for me. Again, I did not understand the seriousness of what was going on, but I knew this needed to be done if Michelle was going to survive. It's not that I thought that Michelle must survive at any cost. I was just swept along with what the doctors recommended. There was no way for me to make a reasonable decision as to whether or not I should refuse surgery. Michelle was entrusted to their care.

Michelle survived the surgery and was immediately put into isolation. This meant that she was taken to a room in the back of the unit where a nurse watched her constantly from outside her door. Everyone who went into her room needed to wear a paper gown and mask and scrub on their way in and out. During this time she also received her ninth pint of blood. Her friends joked that she was probably receiving her own blood because she had donated blood so frequently.

While Michelle was lying in isolation, so much was happening in the unit and the waiting room. On Saturday night, I had heard one of the neurosurgeons inform the parents of a young man that their son was brain dead. I expected to find his bed empty on Sunday but it was not. He was still lying there attached to his ventilator. Again, on Monday morning I found him in his bed. I asked Michelle's nurse how long one is kept on a ventilator after they have been declared brain dead, and she told me that he was going to be an organ donor. On Tuesday morning, I saw a whole team of doctors around him who I had not seen before and heard a doctor on the phone describing muscle density. I knew that this must be the transplant team.

Young people who die of head injuries are the best source of organs for transplantation because their organs are young, fresh, and not riddled with disease. Michelle would be an ideal donor and I knew that Michelle would want to be a transplant donor, but I had an intense need to hold her in my arms without any tubes attached should she die. She was my daughter. I knew I would not need to do this if it were my husband or mother who died, but my child was a different story. This urge was so strong that I agonized about this decision for days. I had never read about it in any of the ethics books, but I was haunted by it. Do I do what I need to do to remain psychologically whole, hold my daughter in my arms without tubes, when in the process I might be denying others needed organs? Or do I sacrifice my well being for the good of others? Organs need to be fresh for transplantation, and I wasn't sure how long one could be detached from a ventilator before one's organs would deteriorate. I kept asking Michelle's doctors the time limit, but no one was exactly sure. The image of the Pieta had never been so powerful.

The weekend Michelle was in isolation was also the weekend that two members of rival gangs were in the neuro ICU. This meant that I was sitting in the waiting room with their family members and friends. One could see the hatred on their faces, especially on the face of the young brother of one of them. It was necessary for the hospital guards to come and remove most of them from the waiting room. I was relieved.

It was also around this time that Dorothy's daughter – "fast mama," as Dorothy referred to her – was being released from the hospital. Dorothy was a waiting room regular, who showed up early every morning to be with her daughter who was recovering from an operation to remove a brain tumor. Dorothy approached me and asked if she could ask me a question. She started by saying that she knew I was smarter than she was, and she wanted to know if her daughter had one of those things in her head like the boy who kept returning to the hospital and Michelle. I knew she meant a shunt, and I realized that she didn't know the word to describe it and could not ask the doctors. I told her that her daughter did not have a shunt, and she burst out in tears and thanked me. She must have been observing the turmoil that we were going through every time Michelle's shunt became infected and did not know whether her daughter also had a shunt.

Around this time I also met Ginny, who is related to the person who was at the time mayor of our village on Long Island. She was a nursing professor at Rush Presbyterian Hospital, which is next door to Cook County Hospital. Our mayor, Claudia, had told Ginny of Michelle's accident, and Ginny began to visit us every day at Cook County. She would spend time with us, check up on Michelle's care, and offer us all kinds of support.

Ginny was with me the evening that I was sure Michelle was dying. Michelle was still in isolation and was visited every day by doctors of infectious diseases. As I walked into her room Friday evening, March 20, I became convinced she was dying. Her ventilator read mandatory for several hours. The doctors could evoke no pain response from any part of her body, and there was blood flowing from the shunt in her brain into the external bag. I was so panicky that I forced the nurse to call the doctor to let him know that Michelle was dying. It was difficult for him to reassure me because I know he thought that she was also. There was nothing any of us could do but sit and wait.

While we waited the several days until Michelle recovered from this latest crisis, relatives were still flying out from New York to be with us in Chicago. My sisters-in-law Corinna, Chrisy, and Donna came, as well as my nieces Suzanne and Laura. My husband and sons kept flying back and forth, Michelle's friends from Chicago continued to visit, and her resident heads, Paul and Pushpita, were with us every day. I had tremendous support, which I know is what carried me through.

During this time we also were interviewing lawyers, and I was attempting to find out where Michelle stood academically. I knew that no matter how this turned out she would never be able to finish the two or three weeks that she had left of this quarter at the university. I asked her advisor, Jean, who visited regularly, whether she could contact Michelle's professors to see if she had done well enough in her classes to pass without taking her exams. If so, she could get credit for the work she had done. Who cared about her GPA (grade point average)?

Events in the waiting room continued to offer momentary distractions from our worry over Michelle. Prisoners were brought to Cook County, so several times a week I would see someone walking down the hall in shackles. One evening a man came into the waiting room and sat down on one of the chairs and began to moan. I asked him what the problem was, and he told me that he had a bullet in his back. He had come to the hospital several times for surgery, but when the doctors told him that a possible side effect was paralysis, he would change his mind and leave. The doctors had refused to give him pain medication because he needed the surgery, so he was roaming the halls looking for someone who would give him morphine.

In the ICU unit, people continued to die. The elderly Hispanic man never regained consciousness, developed pneumonia, and died. The scene was always the same. Family members would gather around the bed to say their final farewell and then the next time I entered the room there was an empty bed, but not for long. Soon another patient would arrive. I had already seen four or five people die.

Michelle did not succumb to the infection. She was finally able to have the shunt internalized and was moved back into the large ICU unit. We continued to wait for her to wake up and worked intensely to have her accepted into RIC. The staff at the hospital wanted her to go to the County Rehabilitation facility. This is where they automatically directed all their patients. But I refused to allow this. As a result, I received little help from hospital staff. They did contact the admission staff at RIC who needed to do an evaluation of Michelle, but now insurance issues began to arise. All I knew was that I wanted Michelle at RIC, and I was like a pit bull in my determination. I refused to consider any options because I felt if I gave the staff any indication that I was wavering they would not help me. I called everyone I could think of to help me–university officials, Sister Sheila, even Leon Kass, a professor at the University of Chicago who had come to visit Michelle.

RIC told us that they would not accept Michelle while she was on a ventilator, so the surgeons began to wean her from the ventilator, and on March 31, the ventilator was disconnected. The nurses also began to put her in a cardiac chair for several minutes every day. She was still connected to monitors so I could see that just sitting in a chair raised her heartbeat to aerobic levels.

The daughter of the woman who ran the elevator, the same woman who brought me fried chicken, was also in the neuro ICU unit, and at one point her mother told me that she was going to fight for her daughter the way I fought for mine. But I knew she couldn't. She didn't have insurance. Without insurance, RIC won't accept you. Although I was accepted by the people who relied on Cook County for care, I understood that I did not experience Cook County the same way that they did. I had options. I spoke English. I was highly educated, and I had many influential people helping me. I had no qualms about questioning the doctors; many others did not have the vocabulary to even vocalize their concerns. I could opt out of the system; they couldn't.

This experience highlighted for me the importance of context when making ethical decisions. Until recently the reigning model of moral decision-making was one that was made from an abstract, universalistic, God's-eye perspective. In other words, the right act was the one that was impartial and capable of being universalized. Desires, inclinations, feelings, etc., had to be left out of moral decision-making because they could easily distract one from doing what was the right thing. To be a moral agent meant that one was not concerned with external ends but rather with doing only what a purely rational agent who had taken the moral point of view, acting from duty, would determine was the right thing to do. Moral agents, therefore, became disinterested, detached, impersonal agents who were motivated by duty and doing what was considered right. Special relationships such as those between parents and children were not considered part of the moral realm but were placed in the realm of prudential reasoning. Family arrangements were not part of the moral and political realms because they involved particular connections between particular persons.

Much of post-modern, feminist, and virtue ethics approaches to moral decision making have called this stance into question. It became obvious that by removing our emotions, attachments, and desires from the moral realm we were distancing ourselves from large areas of our everyday living. Feminist theorists, for example, have stressed that there is no transcendent reason separate from embodiment and time and place. The ideal of normative reason as transcending all perspectives is both illusionary and oppressive. What has become important is the concrete and historical.

However, taking the concrete and contextual into consideration brought me back to my previous concerns of justice. We have become aware of the injustice in our health care where those with the financial resources can get the best health care available while those with little money can frequently not even afford the basics. So here I am in a situation where I am fighting tenaciously for the best care for my daughter while being surrounded by others who cannot afford that care. It forced me to ask myself if I was I demanding more than my fair share for my daughter. I found myself caught up in two contexts, which forced me to think of things I had never thought of before. When sealed in your own context it is too easy to think that this is the way that the world is for everyone. Having spent weeks in Cook County taught me that was not the case. I searched my training for ways to think about this.

Although the ethical literature discusses these issues in terms of parental obligations, I never thought of caring for my daughter in those terms. I never doubted or questioned that I needed to care for her. She was my daughter. There were bonds attaching us. She was in need, and I was her primary caregiver. It was only natural that I would continue to do what I had done for so many years. I thought about these issues more in terms of how do I order my love and concern for Michelle with my other responsibilities? How do I best love my children, husband, and other family members, while at the same time recognizing my responsibility to care for strangers? As far as balancing her overwhelming needs against the needs of my other children, I have reasoned that my sons are adults and capable of receiving less attention from me. (Perhaps even grateful to receive less attention.) In addition, I have said to each of them as they have watched me care for Michelle, that I would be doing the same for them if they were in similar circumstances. Likewise, my husband is an adult and the father of Michelle. He too must be willing to forego some of my attention. I hope they understand.

I did try, however, to think of the others in Cook County Hospital. Perhaps, the best example concerns our decision to stay at Cook County Hospital. We were bringing scarce resources, insurance money, to the hospital. I reflected on Karen Lebacqz's comments in a paper she presented to The Society of Christian Ethics on intersexuality and the politics of difference. A central theme of the paper was whether parents should permit their children to suffer for the sake of a vision or ideal or conviction about society. In her presentation, she highlighted that in efforts to bring justice to an unjust world, suffering is sometimes required. She went on to show how raising a child as intersexed was a just cause and how the suffering these children might undergo was not unbearable.

The cause with which I was concerned was a more equitable distribution of health care. Should I leave the poor simply because I had insurance and could enter another system, or should I allow my insurance dollars to be used to help the poor? I was not willing to sacrifice my daughter's life for this cause – this would have been an undue burden – but I was willing to take some risks and sacrifice my comfort in order to remain with the economically poor. Michelle had now developed two shunt infections during her stay here and I am haunted as to whether these could have been prevented if I had taken her somewhere else. On the other hand, there is no guarantee that she would have fared better in another hospital.

Because of my human finitude there is only so much that I can do. I will never forget these individuals at Cook County Hospital who couldn't get the resources for their family members that I acquired for Michelle. So I resolved to write, lecture, research, and teach about these issues in the hope that others who do not have the support systems that I have will benefit in some way. I hope that by living my particular story the best that I can, social consequences will follow that will benefit others. This is not the perfect solution but is the best I can think of right now.

Thinking in contextual terms also raised another issue for me. If we use an impartial perspective in distributing health care, then the age of the patient should not be taken into account. Much of medical ethics holds that patients should be treated according to strict medical needs and that age should have no influence on their treatment. Because of my profession I have thought about end-of-life issues a great deal, but I have always thought about them in terms of elderly patients who had lived full lives. Now I was faced with the possible death of a young woman, my daughter. This situation seemed so different from the way I had originally thought about these issues.

For a young person, life plans still lie ahead. Despite their injuries, young people's bodies still have vitality and resilience, because the declining biological process associated with aging has not yet begun. It is difficult to describe the conclusion of life for young patients suffering from a terminal illness or injury in terms of a "fitting end" or "dignified death" because their deaths are premature and untimely. There is a terrible waste of potential when young lives that have so much to offer are called to an end. Acceptance is so much harder, because the conclusion of life seems so unfitting in this context.

Should the age factor then be taken into consideration when distributing health-care resources? Should my twenty-one-year-old daughter receive more aggressive treatment than the eighty-one-year-old man lying next to her? Or, because I have special attachments to my daughter, perhaps I should think in different terms. My actual situation provided the scenario for this ethical reflection. As mentioned, the day before Michelle was hit by a car, my father-in-law, Nicholas, had a major stroke. As we flew to Chicago, he lay in the intensive care unit of North Shore University Hospital in Glen Cove. The following Thursday, as Michelle was put into a barbiturate coma to help reduce the swelling on her brain, my father-in-law died. It was on the day of my father-in-law's funeral that we were told that Michelle had survived the initial injury. Intuitively, the family, even my mother-in-law, Laura, felt that if one life could be spared it should be Michelle's. Why?

Perhaps one reason is the symbolism involved. We can imagine a good death for an eighty-one-year-old, but it is hard to imagine a good death for a twenty-one-year-old (especially someone who was so vital only a short time ago). Young people are not supposed to die, at least in our historical and cultural experience. Their deaths seem premature and untimely. This of course works on the assumption that there is a biological progression to life. We move from youth to middle age to old age to death. This is the way we plan our lives as if there is a natural life span. We know that death is inevitable but assume that it will come after a certain number of years lived. We are shocked when death does not follow this timetable. A comment I heard over and over again from family members in brain injury units was, "we knew these things happened, but we didn't think they happened to us." Yes, we know young people die, but for most of us that is a distant thought.

Death represents a break in relationships and we usually think of losing our parents and what life will be like without them, but we don't prepare ourselves for the loss of our child. All our children will die but we usually think that we will not be there to experience their deaths. The death of a child is not a central experience for most people, and society does little to prepare us for such an event. Hence, when the possibility of losing a child arises, our sensibilities are shocked. Something seems totally out of kilter. This should not be.

I do think that age should play a role in determining care. I heard that when Michelle arrived in the trauma room there was some debate as to whether the staff should operate on her because her condition was so dire. They decided to proceed with the operation precisely because she was only twenty-one and they were willing to give her a chance that they may not have given to an eighty-one year old. This is because there is a greater chance that a young person will survive the surgery. This was especially true in my daughter's case. All her other organs were in excellent shape. She had a strong will and high cognitive powers, as well as a great desire to live. On the other hand, my father-in-law had already undergone various other surgeries, was inactive, and was coming to the end of a long and fruitful life. The benefits of extending his life were much fewer than the benefits of extending my daughter's life, so the risks one should take for his welfare should also be fewer. When one is nearing the end of life, palliative care becomes as important if not more important than high-risk procedures. My daughter had multiple brain surgeries. Multiple brain surgeries for someone in my father-in-law's condition would have been immoral. I am not trying to say that a young person's life has more value than the life of an elderly person but I am suggesting that the treatment plan should differ. We should never stop giving care but age should help determine what is appropriate care. But I personally need to be very careful when I speak of the elderly because even though I was gracious to the woman who hit Michelle I will always remember that it was an elderly woman who did this to my daughter.

Finally, on April 3rd Michelle was accepted at RIC. She still was not awake, but we kept hoping it would happen before she was discharged. We were now constantly negotiating with our insurance companies. We needed to wait until a bed became available at RIC and until our insurance had approved the move.

In the meantime, we tried to do everything we could to awaken Michelle. She wore headphones as we hoped that her favorite music as well as Mozart and tapes that friends and family members had made for her would rouse her. Aunt Noreen had sent out a box of scents, and we continually placed various scents under her nose. We sang to her, read poetry, stroked her, but she continued to sleep.

On April 8th she had surgery to replace the naso-gastric tube that fed her. She now had a gastrostomy tube placed in her stomach. This was another sign that the staff was thinking that Michelle's unconsciousness would be long term. I was not ready to think that way yet. My focus was to get her out of Cook County and move on to rehabilitation. How could she awaken when they kept doing surgery after surgery on her? Easter was quickly approaching, and we were hoping for our own resurrection.

On Holy Saturday, April 11th, I arrived at the hospital around 9:00 am. About 9:30, Helen, one of the patients, who was in the bed across from Michelle, got out of bed and was walking around. When the nurse approached her and asked what she was doing, Helen raised her arm and struck the nurse on her head with a metal bar. No one had seen her, but she must have removed the metal bar over her bed that was meant to hold IV bags. The nurse began to stagger and went to the front of the unit while Helen began to race around the room looking for an exit. I stood by Michelle's bedside making sure Helen did not hurt my daughter. But then Helen approached me. I backed her away from Michelle's bed and backed into a corner and stood very still. Helen stared at me, raised her arm and I knew that I too was going to be attacked. But then Helen was distracted by the nurses at the front of the unit and went chasing after them, waving her metal bar. Now I was alone in the ICU. I went around consoling patients who were conscious and had seen the attack. I tried to see if I could secure the door so Helen could not reenter. Soon security ran down the hall where Helen had gone. Now I was shaking. I kept thinking of that look in Helen's eyes. In a few minutes, security and the nurses returned. I asked them where Helen was, and they told me that she had jumped out the window in the back room of the third floor. Security was on the way to get her from the front sidewalk. Just then, my husband came into the unit. He must have entered the hospital between the attack and the jump. With our luck, I found it amazing that Helen did not land right on top of him when she jumped. I began to cry. This was the first time I cried. Up until now I had kept my emotions in check and had focused totally on caring for my daughter. All the excitement in the waiting room, the constant emotional roller coaster with Michelle, and the continued support and caring of others had kept me going. But this was too much. I had reached my breaking point. It was time to get out of Cook County. I did not think I could take much more, and that afternoon I took my first tranquillizer.

Because I was the only one who had actually seen the attack, I was also the main witness for the police investigation. In the evening, Helen was back in her bed next to Michelle. She had only broken her arm in the fall and was still intent on getting out. Now she was in restraints and a nurse sat by her bedside, but she still had that frightening stare in her eyes. I asked the nurses to have her put in the psychiatric unit. I was so afraid that she would hurt Michelle. They told me that I had to understand that she had a brain tumor and could not be held responsible for her actions. I responded that I was not trying to allocate moral guilt but only trying to protect my daughter. Easter arrived, Michelle slept, and I ate hot dogs for dinner from the greasy spoon across the street. So much for our resurrection.

Finally, Wednesday morning, April 15, we received word that a bed was available at RIC and we were going to be transferred. Alleluia! Larry contacted the hotel near RIC that was holding our room and then began packing up our belongings from our hotel room. He made the move to the new hotel and went to RIC to do the paper work and get things set up there. I sat by Michelle's bedside waiting for the ambulance to arrive and transfer us to our next destination. Michelle slept.

When the surgeons at Cook County said goodbye, they told me that Michelle had years of rehabilitation ahead of her, and I told them that there was one tough woman in the bed and one tough woman beside the bed. We would do this together.

I determined that Michelle needed to be treated as Michelle and not as some nameless, interchangeable human being. Her care depended on the proper assessment of who she was. I realized as we left Cook County that it was now my responsibility to keep her story alive. Who she was before the accident and what happened at Cook County would be reduced to short, bland discharge notes. My role evolved naturally into keeping Michelle's dignity and personhood in tact. She was more than a twenty-one-year-old female who suffered from a head injury. She was Michelle Martone, a bright, funny, compassionate young women who had worked endlessly to try to make the world a better place to live.

After an emotional farewell to the staff, who had taken such good care of Michelle, the patients, and my friends in the waiting room, we left. I climbed in the back of the ambulance with Michelle, knowing that there was little I could do to bring her back to consciousness, but I could try to make sure that no further harm came to her. I could be her storyteller, her decision maker, and her guardian. I hoped that I was up to it.

We went cross-town to RIC after spending seven and half weeks at Cook County.

4.

Rehabilitation Institute of Chicago (RIC)

When the ambulance arrived at RIC, Larry was waiting for us. The paperwork had been done so we were taken directly to a room on the eighth floor. The staff transferred Michelle from the ambulance stretcher into a hospital bed. It was strange for both Larry and me because Michelle was no longer attached to any machines that told us numbers. We had nothing to watch. In the hospital we had become fascinated with numbers. First it was the intracranial pressure number; then we were fixated on ventilator numbers and after that blood pressure, heartbeat, respiration, etc. Now there were no numbers to watch.

Soon the doctor came to examine Michelle. I was ecstatic because we were finally out of the hospital, and I was convinced that now that Michelle was medically stable, and would hopefully not undergo any more surgeries, she would wake up and begin her recovery. I had a comfortable place to stay, and I was even planning on going to the gym in the hotel every day and begin to have some semblance of normalcy in my life. But the doctor soon shattered those hopes. After he had examined Michelle, I asked him for a prognosis. He turned to me and said that I needed to remember that she had suffered trauma not just to one side of her brain but to both sides, and I should not expect too much. At Cook County Hospital the staff told me to pray for miracles. Faith and hope exuded from the hospital even though I thought I was looking only for good medical care. When Michelle was finally admitted to one of the best rehabilitation facilities in the country, one that had an entire floor devoted to head injury, we were welcomed with news that held little hope. What I was looking for was a balance of the two – not false hope, but the possibility that the human brain might be capable of much more than the doctors could predict.

Right after the doctor left, my chairperson from St. John's, Jean-Pierre, walked into the room. He was in Chicago for a conference and stopped in to see me. I remember turning to him and crying and telling him that the doctors did not give Michelle much hope. I'm glad he walked in before my husband because I wasn't sure I could tell Larry what I had just been told.

I met many people that day. It was a strange feeling walking through the halls. There were many windows in the building and one side faced Lake Michigan. What a beautiful sight to sit in the large common room and look at the lake. But some of the sights and sounds coming from the patients' rooms were frightening.

I had as my reference at this point only the TV image of what a person looks like in a coma and how a person *awakens* from a coma – the person's eyes slowly open and he or she may even whisper "hello." This was very different from the reality I was soon exposed to. As I walked the halls of RIC, I soon learned that one could have one's eyes open, move, and even groan and still be unconscious. I also saw others emerging from unconsciousness. I saw mesh beds that looked like large playpens that were zippered all around with people in them jumping, screaming, and moaning. There were other individuals with all kinds of splints on them, propped up in wheelchairs and drooling. Others were cursing wildly. Some were walking around with glazed looks in their eyes, not sure where or who they were. But there were also others who seemed to have made miraculous recoveries and would soon be going home.

As the days passed, I was desperate to learn what could be done so that Michelle could be one of those who would recover and go home. I was told that if Michelle did not awaken in two weeks and begin rehabilitation in earnest she would have to leave. The institute could not justify keeping her longer than that. Trying to rouse Michelle out of a coma required refraining from overstimulating her brain while knowing that if she did not show signs of consciousness within RIC's narrow time frame she would be discharged. This was my first introduction to the concept of *plateauing*. If a patient does not recover at a sufficiently fast rate, the patient is said to have plateaued. In other words, RIC had determined that they could only justify a two week stay for those who are unconscious. Once someone does emerge from unconsciousness they need to show continual rapid progress in order to stay in a rehabilitation facility. I found this concept very strange. To me it seemed like the system had it backward. If something wasn't working why wasn't more or a different type of therapy added? Why was the patient always the one at fault? Plateauing focuses on the patient's inability to meet goals that have less to do with the patient's condition–particularly in the instance of brain injury–and more to do with the allocation of resources. It also does not judge the competency of the health care professionals and the facilities in which they work. Rather, this approach makes it possible for institutions to improve their outcomes by directing most of their resources toward patients who show the greatest chance of recovery in the shortest time. It's a self-perpetuating system because admissions to highly rated rehabilitation centers are highly selective – the facilities accept and retain the patients who have the greatest chance of rapid recovery. This means that the most severely injured patients are denied rehabilitation, and those who need more time to recover are denied assistance. Furthermore, if families accept the concept of plateauing, they may give up on their loved ones sooner than they should. On the other hand, if a family is told that their loved one has plateaued and then later that person makes significant progress, family members lose trust in the health-care professionals. Caring health-care professionals are also constrained by this system and are forced to write very creative notes to insurance companies so that services will not be cut. I was learning that there is a strong emphasis on acute care and fast recovery in our health-care system and few resources for those who have chronic conditions.

Where would Michelle go if we were forced to leave RIC? I could not imagine putting my daughter in a nursing home. She was twenty-one. Several weeks ago she had been a vibrant, brilliant young woman. Now it seemed as if no one wanted her. Were we going to be abandoned by the health-care system? They had saved my daughter's life but now that she wasn't fitting into their structural time frame we felt like unwanted guests. I had so much to learn. How could I best protect my daughter?

Michelle had her therapies every day even though she did very little. In rehabilitation facilities, however, the patients are dressed and gotten out of bed every day. Her friends had brought some of her clothes from her dorm room for her even though many hung from her because she had lost so much weight. Michelle was fitted for a wheel chair and spent several hours every day sitting up in a reclined position. She was still connected to oxygen so we had to move the tank with us everywhere we went. Her foley catheter was also removed, and she was put into diapers. Every tube that left her body meant one less possible source of infection,

My son Larry arrived. My husband had gone back to New York. He was trying to recover from the death of his father and run a business at the same time that he was traveling back and forth to Chicago. In addition, he was handling all the insurance issues of Michelle's recovery and was dealing with the attorney we had hired to initiate a lawsuit against the woman who had hit Michelle.

While we recognized that this was a terrible accident and that there was no malicious intent involved, we also knew that it would be impossible to care for Michelle appropriately without extra income. We had found an attorney, and throughout the entire process we tried to be as respectful of the woman who had hit Michelle as possible. Even though elderly people who hit pedestrians was a big story in Chicago because there seemed to be a plethora of such accidents at the time, we made sure that Michelle's story did not reach the newspapers. We tried to be reasonable and the woman's family was gracious as well.

While my son was at RIC, we met with Michelle's doctor who painted a bleak picture of her recovery. I asked Larry to make sure that his father understood the severity of the accident. I had the feeling that my husband and many of the people back in New York thought that all we had to do now was wait for Michelle to awaken, and all would be fine. Now that I had spent some time in RIC, I understood how unrealistic that idea was, and the doctors continually prepared me for the worst. I had no idea what the future had in store. I frequently dreamt that Michelle sat up in bed one day and said "Hi, Mom," but I knew that was not going to happen. I also had another recurring dream in which I would hear Michelle but she kept getting smaller and smaller until I had difficulty finding her. I would panic searching for her. Was she leaving us? Were others leaving us? How would all this end?

I was becoming more and more removed from my former life and wanted to spend all my time at RIC and be with the other patients' family members whom I met there. It was too painful to be part of the larger world outside. I'd either eat in the cafeteria at RIC or buy food and take it back to my suite. I couldn't eat in restaurants where others were laughing, talking, and enjoying themselves.

One day, I heard that a TV movie was coming on that evening about Carolyn McCarthy and the Long Island Railroad massacre. Although her husband had been killed, her son had survived and made a miraculous recovery. In fact, he started working out at the same gym that I was a member of in New York. I rushed back to the hotel to watch the movie. I frantically searched for any sign of hope I could find. But soon into the movie I discovered that her son had awakened in a few days, and I lost interest. Michelle had now been unconscious for about ten weeks and everyone told me that the longer she lay unconscious, the worse the prognosis was.

Sitting next to someone who doesn't move or respond, day after day after day, makes you think about life differently. Before Michelle's accident, my days were measured by how much I had accomplished. Now what was important was my presence to Michelle and her presence to me. I did not know whether she heard what I said to her. I did not know whether she knew that many people who loved her surrounded her. Where was she? Was she here or somewhere suspended between this world and another? How does one sleep so long? While she slept, however, I could imagine her waking up and being the same person who went to sleep even though all the evidence around me suggested that would not be the case. There was no doubt in my mind, however, that somewhere in the body of the person who lay before me was my daughter, and the most important thing I could do in this life was to sit by her bedside, which I did for hours on end. Michelle was like Pooh in the *Tao of Pooh*: "While Eeyore frets...and Piglet hesitates...and Rabbit calculates...and Owl pontificates...Pooh just is."

I thought a great deal about the concept of time. Michelle and I had always been fast moving. We made decisions quickly and acted on them rapidly. We had both been impatient with others who moved slower than we did. It was important for both of us to accomplish as much as possible in as short a time as possible. I remembered having said to Michelle the summer before that I felt I had lived every day to the fullest. She responded that she felt somewhat the same way. Our days had always been packed with activities. But all that had changed as Michelle slept, and I sat and watched.

I wondered what we were accomplishing even as I pondered how every other activity seemed pointless.

As I watched the people scurrying along the streets of Chicago, I wondered what they could be doing that was so important. In contrast, I had observed how the server in the hospital cafeteria, who had cognitive disabilities, so carefully focused on spooning out the food. It seemed that as one's choices become limited, one is better able to focus on the present and attain a certain depth that is impossible to attain if one is too busy. In focusing on Michelle as I did, I knew every eye movement and sound she made and every scar on her body. I saw signs that she was still with us, but because I was her mother and an untrained health-care professional, my opinions were not valued. I learned quickly that whenever you disagreed with a health-care professional you were considered to be in denial. Yet, no one had observed Michelle as long and as well as I had.

When we examine what philosophy and theology tell us about time, however, we reach very different conclusions. Quick results are not what are important. There is a depth and richness to time. Usually when we think of time it is divided into the past, present, and future. The present is the only state to actually exist. The past is over and the future has not yet arrived. But even the present is not experienced at the precise time it happens for there is a short delay between the occurrence and our consciousness of the occurrence. These two things are never simultaneous.

But there is an intensity to the moment. Jurgen Moltmann, a German theologian, writes in his book *Science and Wisdom* (Fortress Press, 2003) that: "Eternity in time is a category not of extensive life but of intensive life." This eternity is the depth dimension of the present.

As I sat by Michelle's bedside as she slept, I experienced this depth of time. Many days were like being trapped in the everlasting present yet these days contained much meaning. My total presence to her took me out of the realm of time and placed me in the realm of being.

But we were both in institutions where time could not stop. This was a rehabilitation facility and the individuals who were in this facility needed to produce documented progress. Quiet healing of the brain did not count. There needed to be activity. How much more patient is our God! Modern theological reflection on evolution speaks of God as limiting God's self in order to make room for other beings. And then God was patient, allowing millions of years to pass before life and eventual consciousness emerged. Yet we humans only allow several days for consciousness to reemerge. Moltmann highlights that we have made such importance of the active making of experience over the passive experience of events that objective phenomena can hardly be perceived. If healing was occurring for Michelle she needed time and space for this to happen.

I reflected how the scientific approach to time is somewhat different. Einstein stated that the distinction between past, present, and future is only an illusion. Time is intrinsically flexible, relative, and tied to the individual observer. If Michelle is lying in her bed unconscious of the world around her is time passing for her? Should she awake, will the days that we experienced while she was unconscious have any meaning for her? Will she awake at the same point in time as when she went asleep? I think of the movie *Contact* where Jodi Foster's character visited another realm and met her dead father while those observing her space ship said that she had never gone anywhere and only a few minutes had elapsed.

Whose concept of time was correct? For Einstein there is not universal time or a master clock. Time is relative and depends on motion.

Scientists also point out that our perception of time has something to do with our brain processes. Paul Davies in his book *About Time* (Simon & Schuster, 1995) states if our brains worked at twice their actual speed then one second would seem like two seconds does to us now. So if Michelle's brain is in "safe mode" right now then how is time progressing for her? Or is it? Yet the care that she receives is dictated by our time, not hers. She needs to fit into our categories. Her care is not patient centered but institution centered and institutions cannot waste their resources waiting.

But is there any value to waiting? Is waiting merely passive activity or can there be purpose derived from it? We saw how Moltmann described God's attentive waiting for the evolution of the world. Likewise, John Haught in *God After Darwin* (Westview Press, 2000) describes God as both kenotic love and power of the future. In other words, God is self-emptying love and love by its very nature cannot compel. God calls us and awaits us, while at the same time offering us a wide range of new possibilities.

A waiting grounded in faith, therefore, is not passive. Pope Benedict XVI states that faith is the substance of hope. It is through faith that we believe we have a future and this future is drawn into the present and changes the present. Waiting then is not merely passively existing until the future occurs but engaging the future in the present moment. It is responding to the call of love. Pope Benedict, similar to Moltman, describes eternity not as an unending period of time but a supreme moment of satisfaction, in which totality embraces us and we embrace totality. It is like plunging into the ocean of infinite love where time as we know it no longer exists. How long something takes to occur is not important rather how deeply we embrace the other is what is important.

John Ortberg in *Preaching Today* states that waiting is the hardest part of hope but what God does in us while we wait is as important as what it is we're waiting for. Waiting is part of the process of becoming what God wants us to be. Waiting means that I trust that God knows what God is doing.

It is hard to do this waiting properly when one is constantly being challenged to produce. Appropriate structures, therefore, must be set up that allow us to wait with those who are unconscious instead of forcing us to abandon them. When we are unable to wait, we are unable to hope. We need safe places where we can nourish hope and not merely dumping grounds for those who do not fit into the time structures that have been artificially set up by society. We need safe spaces where we are not alone in our waiting – places that teach perseverance and constancy and give us hope.

Rather than provide me with hope, the social workers and psychologists at RIC prepared me for the worst. They were concerned that I was not processing the facts correctly and that I remained too hopeful. There was no time that I ever had false hope. I recognized from early on that this was very, very serious, and there was no way one could spend hours on a head injury rehabilitation floor without feeling overwhelmed. This was such a profound tragedy that it went to the very core of my being. This was my only daughter, my youngest child, my source of hope and joy. She had promised me that she would pluck my chin hair when I was in a nursing home, and now she was back in diapers. There was no way psychology could help me with this. My goal was not to adjust. I did not want to detach myself from Michelle and recognize boundaries or accept that such an important person in my life could be ripped from me and I should be asked to go on. When people told me that I needed to take care of myself, I would wonder why. How does a mother lose her child and then simply move on with life? But I hadn't lost my child. How could I grieve? If I grieved for what I had lost, it made me feel that I did not appreciate what I had. After all, my daughter was still alive, and she was still my daughter. She was no less than she had been before. But I missed her. I missed her tremendously, and as her friends began to leave her and go about their daily lives, I became fiercely attached to her, guarding over her like a lioness over her cub, making sure that no further harm came to her. While everyone else at RIC was reading *Why Bad Things Happen to Good People* (Avon Books, 1983), I was reading Unamuno's book, *The Tragic Sense of Life* (Dover, 1954) and reflecting on the Garden of Gethsemane. I had no answers, and I had not yet asked why this happened, but I needed consolation – consolation that I could find only in my faith. I needed assurance that there was more to this experience than its tragic weight, or I might have gone mad. My goal was not to adjust but to find meaning.

While I read and reflected on all of this, my family and friends continued to carry me. On April 23, my friend Delia arrived from New York. It was a very stressful day because all day the staff kept talking to me about discharge. I wanted to scream. In addition, Michelle had developed a fever of 102.9. Our attorney also arrived to begin procedures for me to be appointed Michelle's legal guardian. Michelle was twenty-one so I needed to go to court to obtain guardianship of my daughter.

Two days later, on Saturday, Delia and I had spent all morning with Michelle in the common room, and around noon the nurses took Michelle to her room for medicines, her feeding, etc. Delia and I went downstairs to have some lunch. As we were eating in the cafeteria, I heard my name paged, urging me to return to Michelle's room. I thought someone had stopped in to see her and the staff was paging me. When Delia and I returned to Michelle's floor, however, we found Michelle strapped onto a stretcher with several doctors, nurses, and EMT workers around her. I thought that she had had a stroke. They told me that she needed to be rushed to the hospital. Northwestern University Hospital was right next-door, in fact it was connected by an underground tunnel, but when patients from RIC were taken to the hospital they needed to go by ambulance.

Delia and I hopped into the ambulance with Michelle. They took us to the emergency room at Northwestern, and Michelle was placed in a large room between a set of curtains. The doctor came to examine her, and removed a patch on her head during the examination. In the process, she inadvertently exposed Michelle's shunt. Michelle was rushed for a CAT scan, while I followed behind her stretcher. I always went everywhere with her. She was unconscious and could be left anywhere. The transporters only deposited her outside the test rooms, where she was left alone. Anyone could come along and take her, so I stood guard.

After the scan, she was returned to the emergency room, which was now filled to capacity. Michelle just lay in the middle of the room with Delia and me next to her. The male patient who was now in the space that Michelle had occupied kept repeating, "University of Chicago students have the highest rate of masturbation in the country, University of Chicago students have the highest rate of masturbation in the country." Delia and I just looked at each other and smiled. We felt like we were in an episode of "The Twilight Zone."

Michelle was finally taken to a room where the doctor told us that she had pneumonia and that because her shunt had been exposed she would probably need more brain surgery because they were afraid another infection might set in. We needed to wait for the neurosurgeon to arrive. Finally, around 7 pm, Delia and I ran to our hotel and heated up a frozen dinner, and I took my second tranquilizer. It had been a very stressful day. In about half an hour, we returned to the hospital and continued our wait for the neurosurgeon. I was half asleep in the waiting room and Delia needed to be my eyes and ears. I did understand that the neurosurgeon told me that Michelle would need brain surgery to have her shunt removed. It turned out that the shunt was not infected, but they needed to remove it as a precautionary measure. Whenever there was a problem with the shunt it needed to be removed and drained externally for a few days and then reinserted back into her head.

The next day Delia and I went to RIC to remove Michelle's possessions. Now that she was in the hospital, her bed at RIC was turned over to someone else. It was no longer hers. I didn't know what this meant. Was she being discharged? Would we be able to go back to RIC? Or maybe they were expecting her to die. The feeling of abandonment kept growing. The doctors informed me that day that they thought Michelle might have a blood clot, and they began to give her heparin. In addition, her heart was racing, and her oxygen level was dropping.

Delia stayed a day longer than she had planned, but on Monday she left and my husband arrived. The neuro-psychologist from RIC came to the hospital and suggested that we should think about taking Michelle to JFK-Johnson Head-Injury unit in Edison, New Jersey, and I remember screaming at her and telling her that RIC should spend more money on nursing care rather than discharge planning. From the moment we had arrived at RIC, they began our discharge planning. Michelle was in the CCU unit at Northwestern University Hospital with her shunt externalized, her heart racing, her oxygen level dropping, a possible blood clot, and I was told that I should think about going to New Jersey.

Another irony occurred while we were in the CCU unit. Michelle's advisor from the university came with Leon Kass to inform us that Michelle had been elected to Phi Beta Kappa, one of the most prestigious academic honor societies. How should I react to such news while watching oxygen numbers and praying for Michelle's survival? That part of our lives was behind us. I was certainly proud of her but I also realized how fragile life is and what seemed so important just a short time ago now didn't matter. Michelle didn't deserve to be in this condition but then she hadn't deserved to be so brilliant either. It was pure gift. I now had one group of people telling me that Michelle was among the best and the brightest and another group forcing me to get her out of their institution. I couldn't help but feel that now that she was brain injured nobody wanted her.

After several days in CCU, with her shunt externalized, Michelle was returned to the operating room to again have it internalized. We had been hopeful that she would no longer need it, but the CAT scan showed that her ventricles were still enlarged. The surgery went well, but the next day they informed me that Michelle would need more surgery. I asked the doctor why, and his response was that he was human. I respected him for admitting that. They took Michelle to the operating room, and again I waited. Around 3 pm she returned to the room. All had gone well.

The following day, a PIC line (peripherally inserted central catheter) was inserted into Michelle's right underarm because they could no longer find any veins with which to work. They also informed me that we would be returning to RIC as soon as a bed became available. In the meantime, I kept requesting respiration therapy for Michelle. She seemed to have difficulty breathing, and one of the dangers for someone who is unconscious and with a tracheotomy is that she will choke on her mucus. These patients need to be carefully watched and frequently suctioned. It seemed to me that because Michelle was supposed to return to RIC the staff had forgotten about her.

We stayed another night in the hospital, and in the early afternoon of the next day we were wheeled in the underground tunnel back to RIC.

That Sunday was Mothers' Day. What a terrible day! Although there had been very few days when someone from New York (either my sister-in-law Rose, my niece Christina, or one of my sons) was not with me, somehow this turned out to be one of those days. I sat by my daughter's bedside for most of the day, wondering if she would ever wake up, not knowing what lay ahead for her and me. I thought of how Michelle loved children and appreciated her large family. She had many cousins, most of whom were younger than she, and loved to ba-by-sit. When the entire family was together for parties, Michelle was sometimes referred to as "The Pied Piper," because wherever she was there was a large group of young children surrounding her. When she baby sat, she was totally engaged with the children, reading them stories, playing games, teaching them something. She wanted to be a kindergarten teacher so that she could combine her love of learning and her love of children. She often spoke to her friends about getting married and having children of her own. Although her degree from The University of Chicago and her membership in Phi Beta Kappa would probably open many professional doors for her, it was family, children, and the simple everyday exchanges of love that were important to her. Her love of family deepened when she went away to college and saw the many individuals who did not have the same family life that she had. When we returned from taking her to Chicago her first year, I found the following letter Michelle had written to her father and me, which she left under my pillow:

> *Dear Mom and Dad,*
>
> *In my rush to get out to Chicago and to finally be on my own (which has been going on for about 10 years), I may have forgotten to say a few things to you guys that I meant to. Actually, there are a million and one things I would have liked to have said, but I've always found writing easier.*
>
> *I hope you both will always know how much I love you. I thank God so often that I was lucky enough to be born into this household – even more so now that the boys have outgrown beating me up. So many people I know, even close friends, come from messed-up families or "messed-up" in my opinion, anyway. Mom, I know sometimes you wish we were all closer, but I don't think you realize what a good job you've both done. I think in time we'll all grow up a little more, but for now, I couldn't*

be prouder of the family life I've known. I've never in life felt need of something I didn't have and I really don't know how I got so lucky.

I think in this past week I've just started to realize how much I'm going to miss this place: running down the steps to give Dada the "thumbs-up" signal, having to lie to Danny when he calls every 30 seconds, getting my butt in the driveway by EXACTLY 12:30 (Mom – you'll never know), our dinner-time religion debates, and so many other little things that make up my life. I know I'll never find another person whose dissertation relates to every single thing that is going on in every single person's life! I'm definitely ready to start my new life, but I'm going to miss this one a whole lot.

I just have to thank you both for always letting me do what I needed to – even if that meant the "wrong thing" – in order to grow into the person I am today. I am happy and comfortable with myself, and I know I can only say that because it had little to do with my own efforts – I am what you have made me, and I thank you. I also know that I'm not perfect, and I don't expect to be anytime soon. But you have introduced me to the vehicles of getting there: independence, self-esteem, courage, faith, hope, honesty, sincerity, and most important, the ability to giggle uncontrollably. I can honestly say I love my life – every part of it – and I owe that to you. I have always felt I could do anything and you would support me (I'm just sorry that this time "anything" turned out to be one of the most expensive colleges in the country).

Well, by the time you get this, I'll be gone. I'm sure I'll be having a great time, but I'll never forget how I got there. I don't know what the future holds for me, but I'm thankful that I can always rely on my past to pull me through whatever comes along. I love you Mom and Dada.

Missy

As beautiful as this letter is that doesn't mean that everything was always smooth going. As I stared at her lying unconscious in bed I was still smarting from our previous summer's experience. Our family had gone to Europe for the wedding of one of our friend's children. After the wedding Michelle had planned to do a little traveling with a friend of hers who was studying in Paris. However, at the last minute her friend told Michelle that she could not go. I refused to let Michelle travel by herself through Europe and this caused quite a scene. I went with her and one night after she was late showing up where she was supposed to be she turned to me and said, "You think we're close, don't you? Well we're not." It was like a knife went through my heart. She kept telling me how she wanted me to be her friend, not her mother. In some strange way she had prepared me for today. She had put just enough distance between us that I could care for her without going down with her. So here I sat on Mother's Day saying to my unconscious daughter, "And this is what mothers do. Friends can leave."

The next day, my sister, Kathie, arrived. While Kathie stayed with Michelle, I went to the university. I visited with Paul and Pushpita, Michelle's resident heads. Two days after we arrived at RIC, Paul had called to tell us that Pushpita, had given birth to a baby girl who they named Avani Michelle. Paul and Pushpita had been with us practically every day at Cook County. In fact, Pushpita was with me the day the ambulance arrived to take Michelle to RIC. I was so happy for them and so touched that they had included Michelle's name in their daughter's name. Now I saw little Avani for the first time. I also went into Michelle's dorm room (which was exceedingly difficult because it was just as she had left it when she left her room the Sunday night of the accident) and gathered some of her belongings. Pushpita and some of the students offered to pack Michelle's things and have them sent home, but I wanted to first collect some of her more personal items. I gathered her letters, her computer, her address book, and some of the little things that had special meaning to me. I also saw the scene of the accident, and was amazed that Michelle was still alive.

When I returned to RIC, I found out that Michelle could stay three more weeks. Hopefully, her rehabilitation could begin in earnest, but my hope for this was soon destroyed. The following day, Michelle developed another fever. At about 7pm she was again rushed to Northwestern University Hospital. This time, she had a urinary-tract infection and another possible shunt infection. Michelle's shunt was removed and she was placed in the ICU. Kathie and I did not get back to the hotel until about 2am. I was so frightened to leave Michelle but also so exhausted that I could barely keep my eyes open.

The next day, Michelle was taken out of ICU and put into CCU again. I thought that this could possibly be the end. I realized that she was building up an immunity to antibiotics and was certain that an infection was going to kill her soon. I didn't know how much more she could undergo, or, for that matter, how much more I could. I was totally exhausted, and my sister had to return home. After Kathie left, I just sat by Michelle's bedside, leaned over the railing of the bed, and hung my head. Then the most wonderful thing happened. Someone touched me on the shoulder, and when I looked up, I saw my husband. When I had called Aunt Noreen that morning to give my daily report, she had detected desperation in my voice and suggested to my husband that he should go to Chicago. She was right. This was probably my lowest point since I first arrived in Chicago. I was totally exhausted and losing hope. Larry spent most of the following day at the hospital with Michelle, while I stayed at the hotel and rested.

When I went to the hospital the following morning, I found a large black bag in the corner of Michelle's room. Her possessions from RIC were in it. We had not had time to pack her things before we went to the hospital, and I had been too exhausted to go back the following day, so the personnel at RIC had put them in a large garbage bag and dumped them in her hospital room. Now I truly felt like a refugee. It was as if they couldn't wait to get rid of us. They began asking when we were leaving several days after we arrived back from the hospital, and whenever we went to the hospital Michelle's room at RIC was turned over to someone else.

That afternoon, Tom, a member of our parish in Sea Cliff, stopped by Michelle's hospital room. He was in Chicago on business and came to see us with cards and letters from the people at home. It was the perfect visit at the perfect moment. Just when I was beginning to despair, others again uplifted me. I realized that no matter how strong one is, it is impossible to survive a tragedy such as this without the help of others. We are all interconnected. While hospital personnel began to abandon us, or at least that's how I felt, my family, friends and community embraced me. I alternated between hope and despair, and it was only the support of others that kept me going.

On May 18th, Michelle underwent more surgery to replace the shunt in her head, and I prayed that this would be the last time that they would operate on her brain. I followed her to the pre-op room, and when the anesthesiologist arrived, he asked me how they had given anesthesia to Michelle in the past because she clenched her teeth so tightly closed they could not open her mouth. I informed him that she had a tracheotomy. Her hospital gown was high around her neck, and he had not seen the tracheotomy. This was why I was convinced that I needed to go with her everywhere.

I also spoke with Michelle's neuropsychologist that day, and because Michelle was a psychology major I jokingly told her that Michelle was now doing her fieldwork. She responded that it would be a great accomplishment if Michelle ever reached the point where she could take care of herself. I did not need to be constantly reminded of how serious Michelle's condition was. I lived it moment by moment. What I needed was sustenance to go on. Whether hospital personnel prepared me or not, what was going to happen would happen. I needed them to build me up so that when it happened I would have the strength to deal with it. I did not need to be prepared for the worst–the cold medical facts left little room for hope.

Michelle survived this surgery also and was taken to a regular hospital room. The surgeon had told me that an important issue for Michelle was nutrition, and yet I had learned that Michelle had not yet been fed. When I followed up I was told that the doctor had not issued orders for the tube feeding to begin. I asked that the doctor be paged, but he was in surgery so again we had to wait for the feeding. Hospitals are so focused on the big issues like surgery that they sometimes forget that people need to be fed.

At about 8:10 that evening, the fire alarm in the hospital went off. All the doors were closed, and I was sealed in the room with my daughter and her oxygen. Suddenly, I heard the fire personnel running down the corridor. I stuck my head out the door and asked the nurse where the fire was. She answered that it was on our floor. I ducked back into the room not sure what to do next. Fortunately, within a few minutes the matter was resolved, the doors were opened, and after calming down a little, I kissed my daughter goodnight and returned to the hotel. My hotel was only a block away on the other side of the street and all night I slept lightly listening for fire alarms.

A few days later, after another CAT scan and several blood transfusions, Michelle returned to RIC. After every setback Michelle suffered, we seemed always to have a reason to recognize how blessed our family was. We had constant support. Family members and friends traveled regularly between New York and Chicago to help keep vigil over Michelle, and many colleagues, family members, and friends donated to Michelle's fund at Cook County. Even the lead singer from Michelle's favorite group, Moxy Fruvous, called the hotel and left a get-well message on our answering machine. Michelle had drawn so many people to her, and I recognized that it was only in being able to let go of control that I could continue to accept God's will and remain present to my daughter.

The next day, as I was walking to RIC, I passed the homeless woman whom I passed every day. As I said, "Good morning," she told me that it was her birthday, so I went into the gift shop at Northwestern Hospital and bought her some flowers. I had to share the kindness that so many people shared with me. When you feel like you are gifted you want to gift others.

Wednesday, May 27 was a very trying day. The court-appointed *guardian ad litem* was coming to the hospital to see Michelle. In a few days I would be going to court to be appointed her legal guardian. In addition, I was going to go to the university for the honors ceremony for the senior class. Michelle was receiving several awards, and I planned on being there to pick them up on her behalf. It was almost surreal sitting through that ceremony. Here people were being honored for their brainpower, and my daughter was struggling to stay alive. I couldn't help but focus on the fragility of life. Within a moment, all that we think we have, all our independence and self-assurance, can be wiped out. I realized what's most important is whether or not we have established relationships with people who will care for us should this happen.

The next day, Dr. Kelly spoke with me. He told me that he thought the best place to take Michelle would be JFK-Johnson Hospital in Edison, New Jersey. He told me that the research team there was making great strides in understanding brain injury and rehabilitation, and it would be more convenient for us because it was much closer to our home. If we agreed, he would contact some of the doctors he knew there. He also informed me that based on Michelle's CAT and MRI (magnetic resonance imaging) scans, there was no reason why she should not come out of the coma. He is a kind man. When I asked him whether he had any idea what going through this experience was like, he responded that he did not and that as a father he could not think about it for more than a few minutes. I so respected people who told me the truth.

I was ready to leave Chicago. I was tired, and maybe a change in scene might energize all of us. Dealing with a head injury is very difficult. There is so much ambiguity involved. Everyone recovers differently and at their own pace and yet the medical system allows only a small amount of time for this recovery to occur in an appropriate rehabilitation facility, and if it doesn't the patient is sent to a nursing home. I could not send my twenty-one-year-old daughter to a nursing home. For me, that would have been giving in to hopelessness.

During the next week, there was so much to take care of. Michelle had intermittent fevers, suggesting another bout of pneumonia. I was working with the staff to find a plane to fly us to New Jersey, while my husband was in New Jersey checking out JFK-Johnson and working on the admission papers there. I also had to go to court in Chicago to become Michelle's legal guardian. In addition, I began packing our bags for our trip home. My son Nick and his friend Matt were in Chicago and were returning by train so they would take most of my things home with them, while I focused on collecting Michelle's things.

It turned out that there was a problem arranging for Michelle's travel home, which required chartering a jet. Our insurance company would pay for the flight only if we flew Michelle to one of the nursing homes in the company's health-care system on Long Island. I had a choice of four. Because I refused to go to a nursing home, we had to pay for the flight ourselves. The cost was around $6,400. Michelle's grandfather had established trust funds for all of his grandchildren, and we would have to draw down funds from Michelle's to pay for the flight, but we felt it was important that Michelle go to a rehabilitation facility and not a nursing home. I had learned a great deal at RIC, and I knew the importance of rehabilitation. It was not so much that I thought that Michelle needed a rehabilitation center to wake up, but so far she had not developed any contractures or bedsores, and I knew she stood a better chance of not developing any of these in a rehabilitation center.

On June 10 we left RIC. It was another emotional farewell. We were finally leaving Chicago and flying to the east coast. The ambulance arrived at RIC at about 1:30 pm and took us to Midway Airport. A Lear jet awaited us with a pilot, co-pilot, and a nurse on board. There was an area in which to lock Michelle's stretcher and seats for the nurse and me. The pilot told me that we would be flying above the commercial planes, and the flight should be smooth and fast. There was no waiting for take-off. We were immediately cleared and ascended rapidly. During the flight, Michelle needed to be suctioned several times but remained stable otherwise.

When we approached Newark Airport, our pilot was instructed to land on a runway that brought us to the far side of the airport from where the ambulance was waiting. The other planes in the area were then instructed to clear the runway so that we could get through. It was the most impressive thing I have seen. A large commercial jet veered to the right and another to the left as we proceeded straight to the ambulance.

When we got off of the plane, the ambulance staff asked Michelle's nurse if she would be going to JFK-Johnson with us, and when she responded that she would not they told her that she would have to remove the line from Michelle's arm because they could not transport her with a line in her arm without the nurse. The nurse then said that she would accompany us because Michelle had been through enough and did not need to go through an extra stick. I had met some unbelievably dedicated health-care professionals during this ordeal, and here was a nurse who gave up three hours of her time so Michelle would not have to experience another needle stick.

It took us about an hour to get to the JFK-Johnson hospital because of the traffic. When we arrived outside the hospital, I found my husband and our sons Larry and

Tim waiting for us. We had made it. I felt relieved to have at least brought Michelle home. I thought of another of the sayings on Michelle's door: "Of the blessings set before you, make your choice and be content."

We still had Michelle and now we were closer to home. There was still hope.

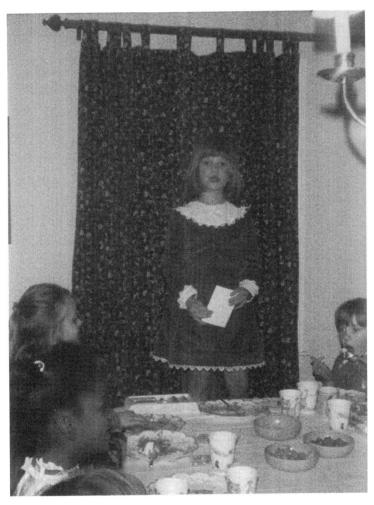

Michelle at her 5th birthday party.

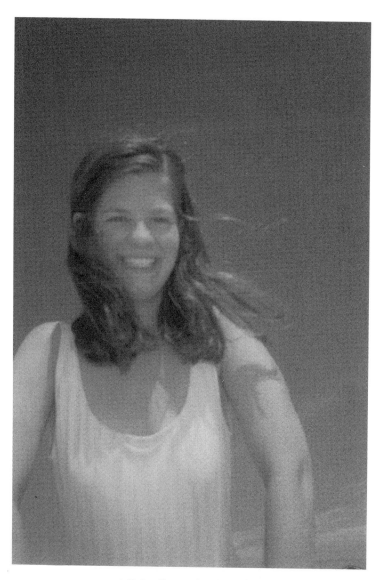

Michelle at the beach.

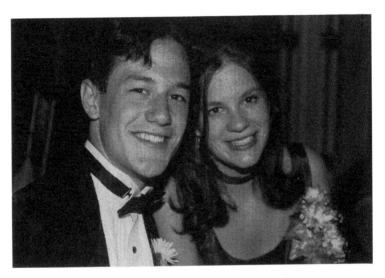

Michelle at her senior prom with Dan.

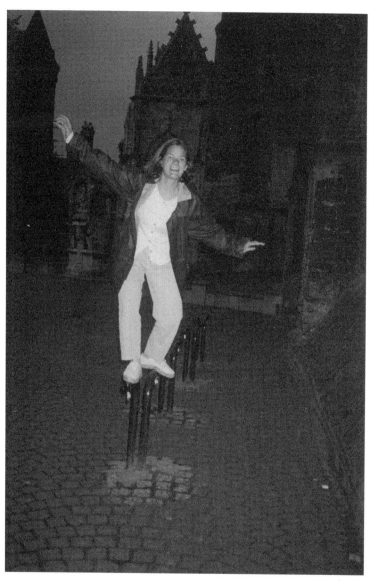

Michelle in the summer of 1997 in Amsterdam.

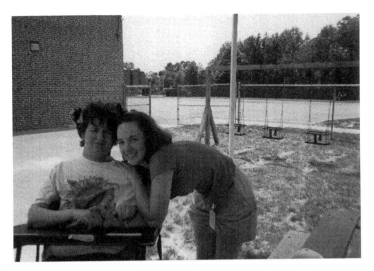

Michelle in JFK-Hartwyck with her friend Kara.

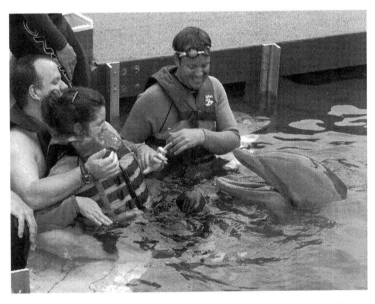

Michelle swimming with the dolphins in Bermuda
with her brothers.

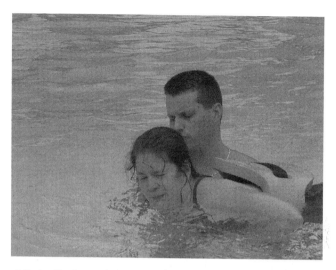

Michelle in swimming therapy with her physical therapist, Doug.

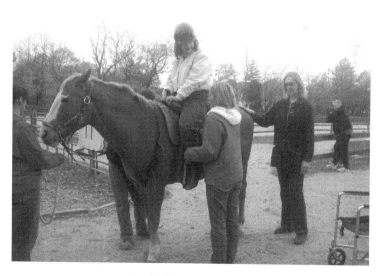

Michelle on Yankee.

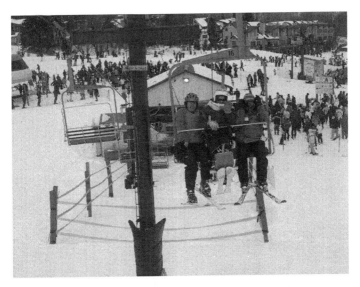

Michelle skiing at Windham Mountain.

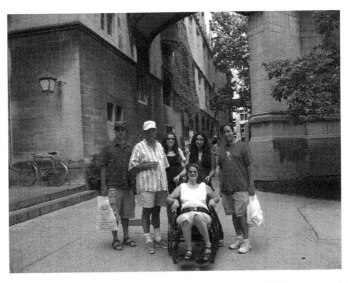

Michelle on a visit back to the University of Chicago with
Dad, Tim and Melissa, and friends JP and Georgia.

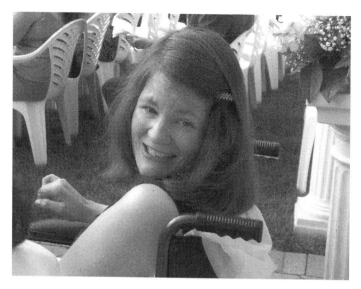

Michelle at her cousin Elizabeth's wedding.

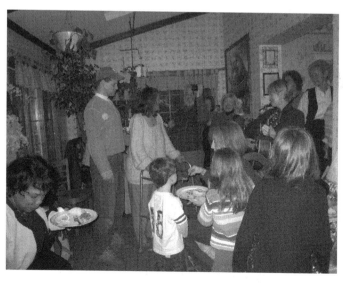

Michelle at one of her holiday parties, surrounded by
many of her therapists and aides.

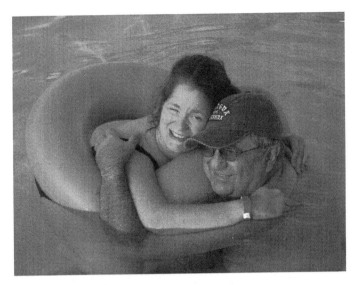

Michelle with Dad.

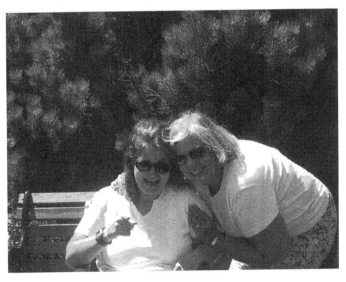

Michelle with Mom.

Michelle surrounded by her family.

5.

JFK-JOHNSON

We arrived at JFK-Johnson Hospital at around 7pm. The nurse who was with us gave her report to the nurses at JFK, and I met Dr. Carolyn McCagg, who would be Michelle's doctor. The staff washed Michelle, did the initial evaluation, and settled her into her room. Finally, around 9 pm, my sons and husband and I left the hospital. Larry and Tim drove home, and my husband and I got a room at a local Day's Inn. They had driven my car to New Jersey, so we now had some flexibility to our schedule. In addition, we learned that the visiting hours at JFK were stricter than at RIC. We could only visit from 4 to 8pm during the week and 1 to 8 pm weekends. In a way, I was relieved. This meant I would now be able to get on some kind of schedule. We also decided that we would now take care of Michelle as a family. This was going to be long-term, so we needed to reserve our resources. I also felt that if I were by Michelle's bedside every day, her father and brothers would feel as if they were not needed, and they were – not only by me, but also by

Michelle. What twenty-one year old wants to have her mother hovering over her every day?

The following day, Thursday, I arrived at JFK around 11 am. I knew that the visiting hours did not begin until the afternoon, but I couldn't wait. It was her first day there, and I needed to make sure she was all right. I met her nurses and some of her therapists. There was an eye, ear, and nose specialist there to examine her, and they also took her for a CAT scan. Later I met Dr. Giacino. Dr. Giacino is a highly respected neuropsychologist who specializes in the vegetative and minimally conscious states. He had done an initial evaluation of Michelle and was cautiously optimistic that she was doing some tracking, which meant that she was following objects with her eyes. She had little reaction to pain, however, and we were reminded that it was now four months since the initial injury, so, although he gave us some hope, we were advised not to be too optimistic. Still, a little hope was better than none. Later that day, some of Michelle's friends, Kara, Diane, and Brendan came from New York. This was another advantage of the move. Now that her friends in Chicago were burnt out we could turn to a new support group from New York, and we needed all the support we could get.

When I arrived the following day, Michelle had just bitten her lip. This was something that she would do occasionally. She would bite her lip, and it was almost impossible to get her to open her mouth to remove the lip. They had tried unsuccessfully in Chicago to fit her with a bite guard, but Dr. McCagg was determined to do this here in New Jersey.

Larry went home for the weekend. We had worked out a tentative schedule whereby he and my sons would each take one day a week to spend with Michelle, and I would take the other three. This way the entire family would be involved in her care, and I would have some much needed time to myself. I also planned on going back to work in September. I was only two years away from my tenure decision at the university, and I hoped to continue my work. I didn't know whether it would be possible to work and to care for Michelle, but I wasn't ready to give up my job yet. I would try this schedule and see whether it was manageable.

Over the weekend more of Michelle's friends came to New Jersey. On Sunday, my brothers, Chris and Kerry, my sister, Kathie, my niece Tori and my mother came from Pennsylvania. It was overwhelming for them to see Michelle for the first time. Her head was still shaved, her skin was filled with acne from the drugs that she was on, her lip was all swollen from having bitten it; she was drooling and strapped into a tilted wheelchair. I was so used to being with her and had seen her so much worse that I forgot how she must have looked to others who had not seen her. My mother started to cry, and I made her stop and told her that Michelle was doing well. I don't know what it was. I would not let people cry around me, nor would I allow myself to cry. It was as if I had a sealed reserve of energy to draw on, and if I began to cry the seal would be broken, the energy would leak out and I would not be able to go on. I needed every ounce of energy I had to protect Michelle. There was no time for self-pity. We were still living in an ambiguous area between survival and emergence. I hadn't lost my daughter yet I didn't have her as I knew her so how should I feel? I'd constantly get fleeting thoughts of how she was.

Michelle was never very concerned with material possessions. It's true she never really was in need of anything, but she never pursued material things either. Her favorite clothes were sweats and sneakers, and the sneakers were not brand names. She took pride in the two plaid shirts she had found in a thrift shop and wore them constantly. She never wore makeup and usually pulled her thick brown hair off of her face, and put it into a ponytail. She seldom wore jewelry, unless it was something that one of her young cousins or someone for whom she baby-sat had made for her. Outside appearances were not that important to her. It was who a person is on the inside that mattered to her. She had bought her little blue Mazda from her brother when he got a new car. She paid her own way on dates, always had a summer job, and saved as much of her money as she could. The quote on her door, "I've learned to seek my happiness by limiting my desires, rather that by attempting to satisfy them" fit Michelle well.

Michelle also loved animals, especially cats. When her friend, Kara's cat had kittens, Michelle picked out a tiny gray ball of fur and named her Buttons. When Buttons was a year old, Michelle and Kara had Buttons' mother over for a birthday party and made a cat food cake for them. But Buttons had a bad habit of attacking birds, and frequently Michelle would take a bird out of Buttons' mouth and nurse it back to health. When Michelle began high school, she got another cat, whom she named Checkers. Checkers was a calico cat and had markings on her neck that looked like a checkerboard. Everyone was afraid of Checkers because she would unexpectedly nip at whoever was nearby, but Michelle referred to these as love bites. Checkers slept with Michelle every night.

Michelle was also known in the family as the mouse catcher. Once there was a mouse running around the kitchen. While the rest of the family ran away, Michelle went over to the cabinet that the mouse hid behind, reached back, picked the mouse up, patted it, opened the back door, and let the mouse run out.

When Kara visited it reminded me that one of Michelle's favorite activities was going for walks on nature trails. She and Kara would often go to one of the preserves close by and walk in the woods. They'd look for animals, bugs, plants, and enjoy their time together surrounded by nature. Michelle could see things on her walks that most other people would miss. She was truly attuned to the things of nature and appreciated everything great and small.

When she graduated from college, she hoped to work for Habitat for Humanity. She had spent a semester break working for that organization and had planned on working there again the semester break right after her accident. Several of her friends had planned on going to Tennessee with her. She loved working with her hands and was always trying to make the world a better place for others. Even though a degree from the University of Chicago would have opened many doors for her, Michelle wanted to do something with her life that would be fun and would help others.

But now how would her life turn out? In the evening, one of Michelle's boyfriends from high school, Dan, came with his parents. Would boyfriends, marriage and a family still lie in the future for Michelle? The medical professionals certainly didn't think so. Michelle remained stable, and late Sunday evening I went home to New York.

I can't explain what it was like to leave Michelle that night. For four months I had been sitting by her bedside for twelve to fourteen hours a day, and now I was driving away. I remember thinking that I would be sixty miles and three bridges away if something should happen. But I also knew that I had not been in control of the situation since the beginning, and I needed to trust the health-care personnel and God that Michelle would be pro-tected. It was June 14, and I had not been in my house since I left the evening of February 22. I snuck in and tried to hide from everyone. For months I had lived in brain injury units. Because the accident happened in Chicago I became disconnected from my previous life. I was not teaching, cooking, doing the dishes, all the daily chores. Nor was I even thinking about daily concerns. I was totally focused on Michelle. From the minute I got up in the morning until I went to bed I sat by her bedside and observed her and others in these surroundings. This had become my entire life. I wasn't sure I was capable of integrating into a world that was different. I had changed. I no longer cared about the things that were so important to me before. It was as if even time had taken on another dimension. I was suspended between the past and the present and had stopped thinking about the future. What meaning could I possibly find in a life outside of these institutions? I desperately needed people to be present to me but I had no desire to be part of their world.

The following day I stayed home while our son Nick went to JFK. I couldn't leave the house. I was afraid some-one would see me. I sent my husband out for some sup-plies, while I just tried to reorient myself. I don't know what I was afraid of, but there was this overwhelming feeling of not wanting to be seen. I felt like a stranger in my own house. Here there were too many memo-ries of Michelle. I couldn't bear to go into her bedroom upstairs or to look at her little blue Mazda in the drive-way. Then there was her cat who seemed to have forgot-ten me. Had Checkers forgotten Michelle as well? Again the feeling of slipping into oblivion overwhelmed me.

I felt like I was becoming invisible just like in the recurring dream that I had had about Michelle. Perhaps I was afraid that if I saw people I was close to in a non-hospital setting I would break down and this was something I did not yet have the luxury to do. I needed to protect my judgment capacities from becoming overwhelmed by my emotions. My emotions were put on a back burner. I wondered how long I would remain like this. One of my friends gave me a book on post-traumatic stress. I didn't read it because I didn't feel I was post-traumatic. This was not a one-time traumatic event but a daily process of trying to come to terms with loss but not sure what one has lost. There was also a sense that if I mourned for Michelle as she was before the accident I would be thinking of her as something less now. But she wasn't. She was still my daughter.

Thus began what would become a daily ritual. On the days that I was not at the hospital, I would call around 6pm to get an update from the family member who was there and to talk to my daughter on the phone. Even though she was still unconscious I was hopeful that she could hear my voice. It was so hard to stay away, but I knew that I had to, and this was my way of still being present to my daughter every day. There was always a family member with her every day to make sure that she was doing well, and I was able to get daily updates.

On Tuesday, I left the house for the first time since I had returned. I discovered that every time I met someone I hadn't seen since the accident, my eyes would begin to well up–I could stop the tears from flowing, but they would always come. Paramount for me was keeping my emotions in check.

The days I wasn't at the hospital I read everything I could find about consciousness. I'm an academic so

I turned to the academic literature. I understood the importance of the brain and recognized that it was the seat of one's personhood. I read the scholarly literature and followed how philosophers and neuroscientists debated about consciousness. Neuroscience has established that our consciousness, which enables us to define who we are as persons, originates in the brain. Although there is general agreement on this, there is still much discussion and much uncertainty as to how the processes that occur in the brain are converted into consciousness. Most scientists agree that there is not a specific part of the brain that is responsible for consciousness. However, disagreement arises over whether consciousness is reducible to solely biological structures. In other words, do our minds arise exclusively from the neurons of our brains? Although some scientists believe that our minds are totally reducible to our neurons and their activity, others suggest that the neurons and the assemblies of neurons of the brain form the foundation of consciousness but that consciousness cannot be totally reducible to neural activity.

The Nobel Prize winner, Francis Crick, believes that our entire personhood can be reduced to the material component of the brain. He refers to this as the "astonishing hypothesis." The astonishing hypothesis, he states, "is that 'You,' your joys and your sorrows, your memories and your ambitions, your sense of personal identity and free will, are in fact no more than the behavior of a vast assembly of nerve cells and their associated molecules." For him, our minds are equated with our brain's neural activity. Our consciousness arises solely from the parts of our brains and how these parts interact. There is nothing over and above this. For Crick, the true description of who a person is lies in the complex interaction of the billions of neurons in a person's brain. (Simon & Schuster, 1994)

Most scientists, however, would argue that science is not yet at the point of having any unified theories of the mind and brain. We simply do not know how consciousness arises, although we do know that we are unaware of about 90% of what goes on in the brain. Alwyn Scott, a mathematics professor at the University of Arizona, likens the activity of consciousness to a ladder, a hierarchy of mental organization. Consciousness is an emergent phenomenon, born of many discrete events fusing together as a single experience. Although consciousness may not be totally reducible to the activity of the brain, nevertheless, the neurons and the assemblies of neurons of the brain form the foundation, or the lower rungs of the ladder, without which consciousness could not exist. Without a brain we could not be conscious. (Copernicus, 1995)

The brain and consciousness are also crucial to our identity. The nuerolgist, Antonio Damasio, describes the sense of self as a private presence, which is directly available only to its owner, and which can be inferred by an external observer only from the influence it exerts on external behaviors, rather than from its own flagship behavior. Wakefulness, background emotion, and low-level attention are thus external signs of internal conditions that are compatible with the occurrence of consciousness. (Harcourt Brace & Company, 1999) Without the ability to communicate with us, without external signs, I had no idea what was occurring inside of Michelle.

As I sat by Michelle's bedside, the scientific debate was less significant than the questions I needed answered, such as, did it matter to Michelle whether I was there beside her? Was Michelle's recovery dependent on passive recovery, or was there something that we needed to do to assure her recovery? Put simply, did we need to do something to jump start Michelle's neurons? While scientists were examining the questions about consciousness in individualistic terms, I wondered about the importance of communal support in aiding brain-injury recovery – does one need others to activate one's brain?

More specifically, I wondered whether Michelle could hear us as we spoke to her, or smell the aromas we put under her nose, or feel us stroke her arms or kiss her toes. Did she see us even though her eyes were not following us? Did she taste the lemon glycerin swabs we rubbed on her tongue? Was she even aware that we were there?

Because I was familiar with some of the stories found in the literature on the brain, I also knew that should Michelle awaken she might be a different person because of her injury. The classic story is that of Phineas Gage. Gage was supervising the construction of a railroad line in 1848 when an explosion blew an iron bar into his cheek and through the top of his head. Gage remained completely lucid and seemed to have little physical damage. Over time, however, those who knew Gage referred to him as a very different man. Before the accident he had been thoughtful and responsible. After the accident he became irreverent, fitful, and used many profanities. His entire personality seemed to change. There are many case studies of individuals who have suffered brain injury and as a consequence develop such conditions as blind-sightedness, hallucinations, neglect of one side of their bodies, anosognosia (the denial of ownership of one's own body parts), Caprgras' delusion (regarding close acquaintances as imposters), and other conditions.

Not only was the literature filled with these case histories, but after spending much time in two of the country's best rehabilitation facilities, I saw first-hand many of the side effects of brain injury. Individuals who were once competent, thoughtful, and independent were now dependent on others to do the simplest tasks for them. Some were in beds surrounded by mesh so they wouldn't hurt themselves, and resembled animals more than humans. The professionals in these institutions prepare you for the fact that your loved one may wake up and have no sexual inhibitions, begin to swear and curse at the slightest provocation, or attack themselves or you. The manual of the Rehabilitation Institute of Chicago, which is distributed to family members of head-injured patients, prepares one to deal with intellectual problems such as impaired alertness, attention deficits, confusion, impaired ability to carry out a plan of action, memory deficits, lack of judgment, impaired language functioning, and impaired ability to integrate new tasks and skills, as well as emotional problems such as irritability, poor emotional control, apathy, lack of inhibitions and impulsivity, lack of insight and denial of disability, self-centeredness, and egocentrism. Depression is also a major concern.

Cathy Crimmins in her book, *Where is the Mango Princess*, describes what it was like when her husband, Al, regained consciousness after a boating accident. She states that he looks the same, although somewhat thinner, but he seems off resembling an alien. (Alfred A. Knopf, 2000)

I had no idea what might lie ahead for us. I accepted the fact that the brain is the key to one's personhood. I accepted that my daughter had suffered severe brain trauma and that she might never awaken. I accepted that if she did awaken she might be a totally different person, but I was her mother and whoever Michelle now was, she was still my daughter. So I would continue to sit by her bedside and continue to stroke her, talk to her, and explain procedures to her the same way that I would have done before her brain injury. Although scientists are uncomfortable with the uncertainty and the loss of predictability that exists with brain injury, it was this very ambiguity that gave me hope. No one could definitely tell me that she would not awaken.

Wednesday was my day to go back to JFK and I couldn't wait. I went with new resolve to be present to my daughter. When I arrived, I found my friend Marge there with her daughter Katie. I also saw that the staff had begun to plug Michelle's tracheotomy, which was a good sign because it meant she was breathing much better on her own. More of Michelle's friends arrived to spend time with her, and I realized how important it was to have people around her so she could be stimulated as well as know how loved she was. On some level I knew that she could sense this, no matter what the literature said. I looked at the man lying in the room next door. No one ever came to visit him, and he just lay there, sleeping all day. We were going to love Michelle back to life. Having others by my side gave me the strength to go on why shouldn't it be the same for Michelle?

Sunday was Fathers' Day. My husband went to see Michelle with his mother and some of his family members, but they had little news to report. On Monday, the social worker informed me that we needed to begin to apply for Medicaid because our insurance was running out. I also knew that if Michelle did not awaken soon we would be discharged to the sub-acute facility of JFK. The staff had planned a family meeting for the following week, and I knew that Michelle's discharge would be the focus of that meeting. Again the fear of abandonment settled in.

I hated social workers. To me they were just discharge planners who were working for institutions that were more intent on efficiency than concern for the patient. I realized that it cost facilities a great deal of money caring for my unconscious daughter but where else could I take her where she would get the same level of care. Everyone seemed to want to discharge my daughter and as medical teams shifted Michelle to different facilities, I realized more and more that we, her family, were responsible for keeping her story alive. In the medical establishment, she was becoming a fragmented person – a successful brain surgery at Cook County Hospital, an unsuccessful coma-stimulation patient at RIC, and a hopeless vegetative patient at JFK. As the medical magic ceased to work, Michelle seemed to become less and less of a person in the eyes of medical professionals. It was up to us, her family, to constantly remind everyone who Michelle was. I felt like The Little Prince when he said, "You know—my flower—I am responsible for her. And she is so weak! She is so naïve! She has four thorns, of no use at all, to protect herself against all the world…"

Our constant presence was the most important reminder, but there were also the posters, banners, and cards that we plastered all over her hospital walls. I wrote letters of thanks to everyone who supported us. Some were published in our local newspapers. As time went on, I wrote articles, many of which were published in scholarly journals. Writing about Michelle was not only a way to help me express what I was experiencing, but also a way to ensure that Michelle would not be forgotten. I was determined to keep her dignity and personhood intact.

Twenty-one boxes with Michelle's possessions arrived from Chicago that week. We piled them into the garage. I decided that I would open them only when she could do it with me. Little by little, I felt that Michelle's dignity was being stripped from her. Her life at the university had been reduced to twenty-one boxes. We had to close her personal savings account and get rid of her car, which we knew she would never drive again. It was all so painful. Someone who had prided herself on her independence was now totally dependent on others for the simplest things in life. It was our thirtieth wedding anniversary that week, but Larry and I didn't even exchange cards. We were both searching for any little way to maintain hope, but we felt as though our world was caving in around us.

After a week or so at JFK, Michelle was put into a room with Sue, who was recovering from a brain tumor. Sue was blind but cognitively whole. It was wonderful for Michelle to have a roommate who cared about her. Every day when we arrived at Michelle's room, Sue would tell us how Michelle had done that night and morning. The head nurse, Debbie, was also very attentive to Michelle. Debbie was one of the best nurses I had ever met. If she did not like the way the aides had washed Michelle, she would take Michelle into the shower and redo the bath. Michelle was medically stable, but was showing few signs of awakening and I knew that it would not be long before we would have to leave. In Chicago, I was fighting for her life, here I was slowly coming to terms with the fact that she might never awaken.

Many of her friends still continued to visit and some even flew in from Chicago. The parish members who began the prayer vigil at our church continued to meet every Thursday night with about fifty people in attendance. This was a wonderful source of support for me.

I watched so many people in the rehabilitation centers go through this ordeal with little or no support; some were single parents, and some were the only support for a spouse. I couldn't fathom what it would be like without the hundreds of people who stood by us. I knew also that on some level Michelle could feel this love.

The dreaded family meeting at the hospital finally took place on July 22. Because Dr. McCagg, who had admitted Michelle, had been transferred to the extended-care unit and because of other demands on my part, we had been able to postpone the meeting for a little while. The team members informed us that Michelle was not improving, and that they did not expect her to wake up. One of the physicians even suggested that we begin to think about withdrawing nutrition and hydration because he believed that Michelle was in a persistent vegetative state (PVS). I responded that it was much too early to think of that, and most of the other team members agreed with me. The physician who was leading this meeting was very blunt and brutal. His attitude was, "you did the best that you could now move on." It wasn't his daughter. All of our sons were there, and after the meeting we went out to lunch and we were all exceedingly depressed. Tim was vehement that we not withdraw nutrition. My husband, Larry, didn't say much, but this meeting would lead to several weeks of depression for him.

The following day I went to the prayer service at our church and cried uncontrollably. The floodgate finally opened. It seemed there was little more I could do. As I contemplated the crucifix, I finally asked God why this had happened to Michelle who had so much to offer the world. As I continued to reflect, I felt that I received God's response: Michelle was not suffering but resting peacefully. I yelled at God and said that we were suffering tremendously, to which I received the reply, "Look around you." And I realized that we had been given lots of support and we were becoming a more loving family and community because of Michelle. From the prayer service, I gathered the strength I needed to go on. My life seemed to be following a pattern that whenever I thought I couldn't continue to go on others lifted me up.

My meltdown showed me the family dynamic that was going on. My sister-in-law Donna said to me afterwards that I was the rock on which everyone depended. When I lost it nobody knew what to do. So I had to be strong.

I also realized that the doctor was wrong and it wasn't time yet for resignation. It was still too early to declare Michelle persistently vegetative, and this was not based on wishful thinking or false hope but on solid medical evidence that concluded that a person Michelle's age who suffers from a traumatic brain injury (TBI) should not be declared PVS until one year post trauma. That was my benchmark. I would wait until a full year had passed before considering giving up hope. But there was the reality that Michelle needed to leave JFK-Johnson and move into the hospital's extended-care unit at Hartwyck. That Friday I went to visit the facility. It was about two miles from the hospital. Dr. McCagg was now the attending physician there so that made the move more palatable. She was very supportive and told me that things were not yet as hopeless as they had been made to sound at the family meeting.

There were forms to fill out, insurance issues, many practicalities that needed to be taken care of. As my daughter continued to be discharged from one facility after another, I continued to look for sources of hope wherever I could find them. The overwhelming feeling

I had throughout this process was one of abandonment. No one wanted Michelle. Because medical professionals and facilities could not fix her, it seemed as though they wanted to get rid of her. We were told that she could spend two months at Hartwyck, and after that we would need to either bring her home or place her in a nursing home. We were able to get Michelle into Hartwyck only because she still had enough money left in her trust fund to pay her way. Because she was twenty-one we were no longer financially responsible for her expenses, and she had not yet been approved for NY State Medicaid, so Hartwyck would accept her until her money was used up and then she would be discharged. There were many compassionate people in these facilities, but they were all controlled by the bottom line.

On Thursday, July 30, we moved to Hartwyck.

6.

JFK-HARTWYCK

Michelle arrived at Hartwyck, the sub-acute division of JFK-Johnson, around noon. She was put into a room with a woman in her fifties–my age–who was vegetative as a result of a brain aneurysm. Ironically, Michelle's roommate was visited by her twenty-one-year-old daughter, who sat by her mother's bedside as I sat by Michelle's, both of us wondering about the recovery and fate of our loved ones. At Harwyck, there were many other patients who were vegetative, and some had been at this facility for long periods of time. Was this the future that Michelle had in store? Many patients could be heard groaning, several were contracted and curled up in fetal positions, and others were lined up in the community room in their tilted wheelchairs staring into space. There were several New York City policemen here. I had also met several policemen at RIC in Chicago, and I came to realize what a price some of these men and women had paid in the line of duty.

I started to go to a support group for families of traumatic brain injury patients at a hospital on Long Island. I went with one goal in mind. I was desperately searching to meet someone who had been unconscious as long as Michelle had been but recovered and was conscious. I met a family at the support group meetings who told me that their family member–Jim–had been unconscious for a long period of time and was now making significant progress. Jim's mother, Jane, called me and offered me significant hope as well as the names of several therapists and programs that had helped her son. But first Michelle had to awaken.

Our routine continued. Nick, Larry, and Tim each visited Michelle one day every week. My husband went on Sundays and I went three days, two of which were usually Friday and Saturday. I would usually spend Friday night in New Jersey so that I could be at Hartwyck by 11 am on Saturday. I had gone back to work, would finish teaching around 2pm, and then drive to New Jersey. Family members and friends continued to visit, and Don and Julie spent every Saturday with me. We were determined that Michelle would not be alone and forgotten.

We were also in the process of applying for Medicaid, which I found difficult to accept. We were an upper-middle-class family, and we had always been financially responsible. Michelle had car insurance and health insurance, she had worked and saved money, and she had the added advantage of a trust fund to draw on. I realized, however, that with catastrophic illness, this was not nearly enough to cover the cost of health care. At the time of Michelle's accident, a one-month stay in an acute-care facility cost about $30,000. Most insurance companies pay for a month of rehabilitation. After that, patients who don't wake up are put into nursing homes. In order to ensure continued rehabilitation care for Michelle, she needed to have Medicaid coverage because her own money was quickly being depleted. It was easy for a twenty-one year old to reach the poverty levels one needed to reach in order to be eligible for Medicaid. There were so many people I met who had to spend down all their available funds and sell property in order to get the needed help for their loved ones. Poor patients in Michelle's condition never get into top-quality rehabilitation facilities, and those who can afford to get into these facilities become poor if they do not make rapid progress. Our system is set up for quick fixes.

We applied for Medicaid because I realized that this was the only way I could get the services I needed for my daughter, but I did have guilt about it because I knew that there were so many others out there who needed the assistance as much as we did and who were not getting it. I cannot imagine what it must be like to be economically poor and watch your child be denied services because of money. I resolved I would do everything I could to try to bring about a more equitable distribution of health care.

It was a very difficult summer. I was trying to bridge two worlds. I was home and semi-functioning in a normal environment while at the same time knowing that my life would never be the same again. How painful it was to go into the florist shop and see a young woman and her mother picking out flowers for her wedding or even being in a restaurant and watching a mother and daughter lunch. Larry and I had bought Broadway play tickets before Michelle's accident for that July and I went to the theater with him because I thought I needed to have some time with my husband, but during the performance, I thought I would go out of my mind. How does one sit in the theater and enjoy oneself when one's daughter is lying vegetative several miles away? This guilt complex stayed with me for a long time. I felt that it was wrong for me to enjoy anything while my daughter was incapable of experiencing joy.

Then there was my trip to Lord and Taylor to buy gift certificates to thank those who had covered my classes while I was in Chicago and seeing a woman from my home town and thinking that she had no idea of what I was going through as she went about her daily routine. Several weeks later her son was killed in a motorcycle accident. None of us know what life has in store for us, but some of us are more acutely aware of life's uncertainty than others.

Meanwhile, Michelle made little progress over the summer. I alternated between hope and despair. There were some days when I thought that she was responding somewhat, and other days when it took every ounce of courage I had to want to stay alive. Michelle's left side seemed to be getting stiffer, and her hand seemed to be getting contracted. I stretched and stretched her, hoping that this would not happen. Splints were made to keep her hand outstretched. Her wheelchair had a headrest with extensions on the sides to keep her head straight. She wore special boots at night to keep her from getting foot-drop. I insisted that she have an air mattress in order to prevent bedsores.

One day when I arrived at Hartwyck, Michelle was in the community room, and I thought that she had suffocated. I saw her wheelchair and her legs but only a pillow at the back area of her wheelchair. When I got closer, however, I saw that she had fallen to the side and was leaning over the left side of her wheelchair. She could not even hold herself up.

I spent all my free time reading everything I could about suffering, added to my readings on consciousness. I started with the book of Job in the Bible and read C.S. Lewis, Peter Kreeft, Jorgen Moltmann, Victor Frankl, as well as the works of many mothers who dealt with the suffering of their children, such as Martha Beck, Karen Brennan, and Ruthann Knechel Johansen. Although the rehabilitation facilities gave you readings to help you adjust and get through this experience psychologically whole, I was not interested in adjusting; I wanted to make sense of this experience. What meaning could there be in having a beautiful, intelligent, kind young woman reduced to a drooling, totally dependent person? But I knew that there was meaning, there had to be meaning, or everything about this life was senseless, and there would be absolutely no reason to go on. In fact many nights when I was driving home from New Jersey I'd think that it made no difference if I got into an accident and died. But then I would return to Michelle's bedside.

Sitting by Michelle's bedside and being present to her was meaningful in itself. However, I was searching for meaning in a larger sense. I wasn't sure what that was, but I had clues. I recognized how Michelle and her story touched others. She was like a magnet drawing out the best in others. She took all of us out of ordinary time and made us stop and reflect on the meaning of life. Suddenly, everything we thought was important–all of our day-to-day commitments and goals seemed empty and insignificant. Instead, Michelle's life pointed to what was really important. Michelle continued to live but was bedridden and barely able to communicate and yet she taught us what really mattered. Our hopes and dreams shifted, and we reprioritized the "stuff" that filled our days. Life was becoming pared down to its essentials even as we continued to be engaged in the daily details. It was a painful but revealing process.

As the noted psychologist, Sidney Callahan states in her book, *Created for Joy* (Crossroad Publishing Company, 2007), when we are faced with mystery we need to go down the road toward comprehension as far as possible. So I tried to understand the full import of our changed circumstances by returning to all that I had read about suffering and what I had learned from the experiences of others. First, I realized that suffering is just part of life. Many people throughout the world are much more willing to accept this fact than we are in the United States because we have been led to believe that we can control everything. There are just some things beyond our control. Aristotle would have called those occurrences, moral luck. What happened to my daughter was a terrible accident. She was just at the wrong place at the wrong time, and it was useless to think, "what if?" What if she had left her room a little later? What if she was standing two feet to the right? What if she had had her car on campus and would not have been waiting for the campus van? She was where she was when she was. She was not involved in any high-risk behavior. She just was there. There was no way to make sense of what could have been done differently. It happened. She was hit by a car and severely brain-injured, and now it was up to us to make sense of the experience. It was not just that our daughter might die, but that her death would be against what we had accepted as the natural order of things, that parents predecease their children. In our case, this might be reversed.

Second, I came to realize that we experience loss because we have something to lose. Each object of loss started as a gift. In the Book of Job, Job's wife says to him,

"Are you still holding to your innocence? Curse God and die." But Job responds, "Are even you going to speak as senseless women do? We accept good things from God; and should we not accept evil?" Job reminds us, "Naked I came forth from my mother's womb and naked shall I go back again. The Lord gave and the Lord has taken away; blessed be the name of the Lord." Everything about us is pure gift. We were not able to bring ourselves into existence or to keep ourselves in existence. Why is it that when good things happen in our lives we think that we are responsible for them, and when bad things happen we blame God? The only reason I was experiencing suffering was because I had been gifted with a daughter in the first place. Many people never receive this gift.

Perhaps the most famous book on suffering is Viktor Frankl's, *Man's Search for Meaning* (Washington Square Press, 1959), in which he describes his experience in the Nazi concentration camps. Frankl highlights that no matter what one's circumstances might be, each of us still has the freedom to choose the stance that we take toward those circumstances. This is where meaning is found, in the way that we bear our burdens. For Frankl, life holds meaning even under the most dire of circumstances.

Frankl states that love is as strong as death, and when we experience love, death loses its sting. Morrie, in the book, *Tuesdays with Morrie* by Mitch Albom (Doubleday, 1997), highlights the same point. Morrie stresses throughout his conversations with Mitch that love is supremely important. Love is how you stay alive even after you are gone, and it is what keeps you going while you are alive. For Morrie, learning how to give out love and let it come in was the most important thing in life.

Frankl and Morrie also stress that as our external world becomes smaller, our interior life grows larger; in other words, there is a greater depth to our experiences as our experiences become compressed. This is what I experienced as I sat by my daughter's bedside. There was no conversation, yet I was able to interpret every movement of her body, movements I would not have previously noticed. Morrie spoke of how he appreciated the window in his room because it allowed him to see how the trees changed, how the wind blew, and other things about nature.

In *Man's Search for Meaning*, Frankl also comments that after all he had suffered there was nothing to fear anymore except God. Although I don't fear God, but think of God more as merciful, I have found that I have developed a similar sense of fearlessness, after surviving the near-death of my daughter. I could not imagine anything worse than the death of one of my children, and yet I was forced to face that possibility that first night in Chicago and many times after that as Michelle suffered one crisis after another. Even now, when I worry about my sons, it is their deaths I fear. I am fearful of little else. Then I remember that I have already come to terms with the possibility of losing a child.

Another consolation in reading about suffering was finding that I had reacted similarly to the way others had reacted to traumatic events. For instance, when Martha Beck describes her reaction to receiving the news that her unborn son was diagnosed as having Down's Syndrome, she writes that she never asked "Why me?" She too recognized that she had had so much good fortune in her life that it was only inevitable that some bad luck would come as well. And as I had felt it was important to assure Michelle that I would be faithful to her no matter what, Beck states that her whole life hinged on knowing that if she were to become incapacitated or sick, she had family and friends she could depend on, who would love her unconditionally. She also stated that after her son's birth she prayed for the first time without trying to control what the answer might be. Throughout Beck's book, *Expecting Adam* (Random House, 1999), it is obvious that Beck views her son as a gift and that love is the driving force of her life.

When I read Karen Brennan's book, *Being with Rachel* (W. W. Norton & Company, 2002), I could easily relate to the description of Brennan's journey with her daughter through her daughter's recovery from a head injury. Brennan questions whether her daughter is in a state that is more real than the reality in which we go about our busy lives. She picks up on Frankl's notion of meaning, stating that the way each of us chooses to look at the world becomes the world that we look at. Brennan states that she vowed that she would always be there for her child, as I had for Michelle and Beck had for Adam.

There were themes running throughout all of these works that directly connected to my experience. But because I am a theologian, I also reflected on these experiences theologically, with the main theological reflection focusing on why we suffer. I had read Rabbi Harold Kushner's book, *When Bad Things Happen to Good People* (Avon Books, 1981), and although I could relate to his argument that God is good but when God set things in motion God more or less stepped back and allowed things to unfold, I had trouble integrating this with my belief that God is all powerful. C.S. Lewis in the *Problem of Pain* (Touchstone Book, 1996), highlights this problem. It is that if God were good, God would want God's creatures to be perfectly happy, and if God were Almighty, God could do what God wished. Therefore, God lacks either goodness, or power, or both. I believed God was good and powerful, therefore, how could I describe human suffering? I knew I was suffering at the most profound level possible and yet I continued to believe in a powerful God.

According to C. S. Lewis, we can ascertain the meaning of our experiences only when we surrender ourselves to God. It involves an appreciation of our limitations and a willingness to accept that no matter what, God loves us and understands what is best for us. Suffering, sometimes, shatters our false sense of self-sufficiency. Surrender to God's will, without totally understanding God's will, is what Lewis calls us to do.

Jorgen Moltman, in *The Crucified God*, (Harper & Row, 1974), explains the cross of Christ as a paradox. After all, Christ's model of unconditional love for human kind results in tremendous suffering and ultimately death. The cross shows us that the more we love, the more we expose ourselves to suffering. But as love makes us vulnerable to experience pain and suffering, it also opens up the possibility of great joy. Christ on the cross, therefore, showed us that the more you love, the greater your capacity becomes for both joy and sorrow: in short, the greater your capacity for life.

The cross does not show us how to escape suffering but how to be faithful in the midst of suffering. While in Chicago, I often reflected on Jesus in the garden of Gethsemane and how he begged his disciples to pray and watch with him. He knew what was waiting for him and wanted companionship and support. I too was more afraid of being alone than I was of Michelle's death. Joseph Cardinal Bernadin wrote in his book *The Gift of Peace* that Jesus did not promise to take away our burdens, but only to help us carry them. We, too, are called to be a faithful people and to help each other carry our burdens. The only promise I made to my daughter was, "I will never walk away from you." All that had transpired since the accident brought me to this place–I found meaning in my presence to Michelle and the community's presence to me.

But that meaning was in constant danger of being shattered. On August 24, Michelle's neuropsychologist, Dr. Giacino, did an evaluation of Michelle. He saw little progress and was not able to determine that she was even minimally conscious, although he still detected some eye tracking. He informed me that she had only a 15 percent chance of emerging from the vegetative state. His conclusion read:

"Based on the results of today's evaluation, she does not show any definitive behavioral signs of consciousness or cognition. There is, however, evidence of recent reemergence of visual tracking, although the trajectory of these eye movements is relatively short and they do not occur spontaneously. It will be important to continue to monitor these eye movements since they often represent an early indication of the transition from the vegetative state to consciousness. There is also questionable active movement of the extremities on the left side but this only occurs subsequent to application of noxious stimulation. Arousal is poorly sustained but improves in response to deep pressure stimulation.

The clinical findings are indicative of severe, diffuse cerebral injury and are most compatible with the vegetative state, although the recent reemergence of visual tracking suggests the possibility of transition into the minimally conscious state.

Given the apparent degree of under-arousal, stimulant drug trials should certainly be considered to promote alertness and behavior responsiveness.

In terms of prognosis, it is likely that Ms. Martone will be left with severe functional disability, although the probability of recovery of consciousness by 12 months post-injury is more favorable."

Things were looking bleaker every day, and I began to look at places on Long Island where we might place Michelle, while I continued to hope that a miracle might occur.

I spoke with the mother of a young girl who was at Hartwyck. Laura regained consciousness after being in a vegetative state for a long period. Her mother told me that Laura's sister had given her a magnetic pillow for her birthday, and two weeks later Laura began to emerge from the vegetative state. I found a company that sold magnetic pillows and ordered one. I was willing to try anything as long as I thought that it would not hurt Michelle. I also bought some CDs of Gregorian Chant for I had heard somewhere that chant was the same wave length as brain waves. Every night when I left Michelle to return home to Long Island, I would leave her listening to chant.

Over Labor Day weekend, Larry and I both went to New Jersey. It was his birthday and we wanted to be together. We seldom went together. In fact, one of the nurses once asked me if we were separated, and I responded no, we were just practical. We wanted Michelle to always have a family member with her, and yet we all needed some rest, so this seemed to be the best arrangement for us. When one of us was in New Jersey one of us could have some time at home. But this weekend we wanted to be together.

On Saturday morning we went out to breakfast and did a little shopping for a birthday present for Larry. I then went to Hartwyck, and Larry planned on coming about an hour later. Soon after I arrived, there was a fire on Michelle's floor. I was in the room with her, and determined that if it were serious I would throw her over my back and drag her down the stairs that were next to her room.

Larry arrived right after the fire trucks, and he was not allowed to enter the building. I yelled to him from Michelle's window telling him not to worry that I was with Michelle. I only hoped that I was strong enough to do this. It turned out there wasn't much of a fire. I didn't need to evacuate, but there were a few tense moments. This was the second hospital fire I experienced.

There were days in September when things seemed hopeful. I thought that I saw more movement, and I even believed that at times she was following commands. Larry told me that she kissed him goodbye. But there were other days when she would develop a fever, and we were all afraid of another shunt infection. It was such an emotional roller-coaster ride.

At the beginning of October, Dr. McCagg told me that a radiologist had looked at Michelle's recent MRI and had told her that there was more damage than Dr. McCagg had thought. I was slowly resigning myself to the fact that my daughter was going to remain vegetative. I also knew, because of my training, that I had no clear and convincing evidence as to whether Michelle would want to continue to remain in this condition with a feeding tube. If I returned her to New York, I would need clear and convincing evidence of her wishes if we ever decided to have the feeding tube removed. In New Jersey I did not need such evidence. As of now, I was not thinking of removing her tube, but should she remain vegetative I knew this decision was out of my hands if we returned to New York.

The day after Dr. McCagg spoke to me about Michelle's latest MRI, some of Michelle's high school friends, Tamara, Kristen, Brendan, Kara, and Don and Julie came to New Jersey to see Michelle. They had all returned home for a friend's wedding on Friday night and came to New Jersey on Saturday. I had arranged a pizza party. They were enjoying pizza, and Michelle was in her wheelchair next to them. Together they listened to some tapes and I thought I heard her giggle. At bedtime the nurses got her ready for bed, and then all of us surrounded her and took some pictures. I was taking a picture of her and I said "smile," and she smiled, but I had been so trained to think of this as a reflexive movement that I forgot about it the moment after it happened.

The following day my husband went to Hartwyck, and when he came home that evening he told me that Michelle nodded her head for him. I was afraid to believe him.

The next day, Monday, when I returned to New Jersey, I arrived in Michelle's room while the speech therapist was working with her. I told the therapist that Michelle's father told me that she could nod her head to indicate "yes" and "no." The therapist began to ask Michelle several questions–Are you a girl? Do you have any sisters? Do you have brothers? Michelle nodded appropriately in response to all of these questions. I was afraid to let myself think about the possibility that Michelle could be emerging from the vegetative state. I remembered that Edith Stein, who did work on consciousness, was being canonized the following week, and wondered whether she played any role in Michelle's changing condition. I knew some of my friends were praying to her for Michelle.

I returned to New York, and my sons went to New Jersey to be with Michelle on their scheduled days. I was not due to return to New Jersey until Friday, and I was dying to get there. But it was important that

Michelle's brothers be there. They had been so faithful throughout this ordeal, and they deserved to share in the joy of seeing Michelle show signs of responsiveness.

These early signs from Michelle reenergized the family, renewed our hope, and encouraged us to take action. We took cards and games to Michelle and pushed her with all kinds of questions. She even began to whisper some words. When I called one evening at my usual time, she whispered "Hi, Mom." I thought I would never hear those words again. Slowly, she began to speak more. Tim called me one evening from Hartwyck. He was very excited. He told me that at one point Michelle looked very angry, and when he asked her what was the matter, she told him that she was tired. She said it twice. Our daughter was coming back. We were elated.

Around the end of October, Michelle got a new roommate, a young woman who was mobile. I think the staff thought it would be good for Michelle to have a roommate around her age. Crystal didn't have any visitors, however, and I was concerned because she kept looking at Michelle and telling me that she was spoiled rotten. When I was with Michelle she looked at me with hatred in her eyes and sometimes she would get the same look in her eyes that I saw in the woman's eyes at Cook County when she attacked the nurse. Although she had an alarm on her bed, she still kept getting out. When I left that evening, I stopped at the Ladies' Room and heard the alarm go off. When I went back to Michelle's room, I saw Crystal standing by her bed. I demanded a room change. The next day Michelle was transferred to another room. People who have brain injuries can do terrible things. I have seen them attack others, and Michelle was defenseless.

On October 28th, I went with my friend Loretta to visit her. Michelle told Loretta that she wanted to go home. It was a great day because we got permission to bring her home for the Thanksgiving weekend. Her 22nd birthday was on Thanksgiving Day that year, and it would be the first time that she would be home in close to a year.

When our community heard that Michelle would be coming home for Thanksgiving, they volunteered the town's ambulance and crew to bring her home. A team of three or four people would drive to Edison, New Jersey and pick Michelle up at Hartwyck and drive the sixty or so miles back to Long Island and then return her to Hartwyck on Sunday. As Michelle began to regain consciousness, she also began to feel pain. She experienced terrible muscle contractions in the areas behind her knees, where the ligaments felt like taut wires. Michelle would often scream in pain. Dr. McCagg prescribed a new medicine for Michelle to help relieve the muscle pain, but then another medicine was needed to help subside the stomach pains Michelle felt, which were caused by the muscle-pain drug. It seemed that every drug that was prescribed to help Michelle provoked unwanted side effects that could be controlled only by prescribing additional drugs.

It was difficult to watch Michelle experience so much pain as well as to watch the slow progress that she was making. When Michelle regained consciousness, we thought she would make steady progress, but some days she did very little and just wanted to sleep. Other days, she was unable to correctly answer any of our questions. I tried to be patient, but it was very frustrating. However, she passed the swallow test at the hospital, which meant that we could begin to feed her foods like pudding and mashed banana.

November passed by quickly. The staff at Hartwyck trained me to do tube feedings, give medicines, turn Michelle in bed, transfer her to a wheelchair, etc. I had to be prepared to care for Michelle when she returned home for the Thanksgiving holiday and her birthday. We were also able to find an LPN (licensed practical nurse), Lisa, to care for Michelle during the night hours so I could get some sleep.

The day finally arrived when Michelle was scheduled to return home for the first time since the accident. Larry went with the ambulance crew to New Jersey to get her. I stayed home to finish the preparations for her visit home. We rented a hospital bed and set up our den as Michelle's room. There were balloons, banners, and stuffed animals. The entire town anticipated her arrival. She received 13 bouquets of flowers, and while she was home she had 130 visitors.

It was a great visit. She knew that she was home. She knew that she was in the den. She knew the people who came to see her. She even blew out some of the candles on her birthday cake. We all felt so loved. Our daughter was home, and our community celebrated with us. The EMT staff told us that they would also bring Michelle home for Christmas if we wished, and we unhesitatingly accepted their offer. Over Christmas, Michelle was home for a week. Again I was the nurse during the day, and Lisa took care of her during the nights. Visitors streamed in and out of the house. One day we had a songfest with all the cousins and aunts and uncles. Cousins Larry Alf and Gunnar brought their guitars, and we all sang Christmas carols for about an hour. Michelle was tired, but she loved being home with her family.

From January to May, Michelle made only a little progress at Hartwyck. We had been trained to transfer her in and out of our car, and we began to bring her home every other weekend. Larry would go to New Jersey on Friday with one of our sons or a friend and would put her in the front seat of the car with pillows surrounding her and then take her back to New Jersey on Sunday evenings. We now kept a hospital bed and a closet full of medical supplies in our den.

During the spring, my days were filled with the usual busyness of doing the household chores, teaching, marking papers, doing committee work, attending meetings, and yet, the most valuable thing I seemed to be doing was sitting by my daughter's bedside and being present to her. There was no great exchange of ideas, no planning of a future, no decision making; we just were. Sometimes I'd climb into bed with her and watch a movie. Sometimes I'd read to her. Sometimes I'd just sit there and stare into space. But there was a sense of peacefulness and a depth of experience in that room that I did not find anywhere else. It was the simple presence of two people, one to another. She knew that I was there and that's what mattered. It was my presence and nothing that I said or did that was important. I missed this the days that I was not there. There was something that emanated from her that gave me the strength to go on. Her father, and brothers, and I came to her for strength. Every day that we spent with her, we left better people. As it says in the *Tao of Pooh*, "To attain knowledge, add things every day. To attain wisdom, remove things every day."

But again I was pulled back into medical pessimism, although in a realm that is guided solely by empirical evidence it would be referred to as realism. Our attorney and the attorneys representing the woman who had hit Michelle came to New Jersey to see Michelle and to take Dr. McCagg's deposition. Dr. McCagg warned me that there was the possibility that things may not be as dire as she predicted in the deposition. Still it was difficult to read. Some excerpts:

Q. Did Michelle indicate to you today at any point that she was in pain?

A. Yes.

Q. And what was being done to her that elicited pain?

A. I changed her G-tube and pulled the bandage off and pulled the tube out and she cried quite a bit during that time.

Q. With what frequency does it G-tube have to be changed?

A. It depends, it shouldn't need to be changed more that a few times a year.

Q. And is this method of nutrition and hydration something you expect to be permanent?

A. Yes.

Q. Do you foresee a point in the future where she can eat in the traditional, oral manner?

A. No.

Q. And why is that?

A. Because the muscles for swallowing are so weak that she doesn't have the ability to physically get enough food and hydration orally. I just can't imagine that she could.

Q. As a result of her traumatic brain injury does she now have cognitive deficits?

A. I'm sure she has profound deficits in terms of memory, of arousal, and attention, of communication.

Q. Were there other improvements in a physical sense?

A. There were fewer improvements physically. She was able to tolerate being out of bed for longer periods of time. We were able to remove the tracheostomy tube and she was able to take small amounts of food by mouth, not enough to sustain her nutrition, but enough to give her some pleasure. She had really no function or movement of her right side. She did have movement of her left side. She had very poor trunk and head control and really very little improvement in those areas, some, but not dramatic, so she essentially remained completely dependent for all mobility.

Q. Having treated her for about a one-year period are you of the opinion that certain deficits are in fact permanent?

A. Yes.

Q. Do you have an opinion to a reasonable degree of medical certainty as to whether the cognitive deficits are permanent conditions?

A. I believe they are permanent.

Q. How does Michelle communicate? Is her communication limited to mouthing words and somehow gesturing facially to you?

A . Yes.

Q. Is it your expectation in the future that she might form a sentence or is her inability to do so now in your view permanent?

A. She might get better with that, but I think she's going to probably need some form of amenative communication. I don't think it's going to be functional.

Q. You don't see a time, do you, where Michelle will be able to transfer on her own?

A. Oh, no.

Q. That was not very artfully put. So in the future if Michelle is not in bed, you foresee her in a wheelchair. Correct?

A. Yes.

Q. Do you have an opinion as to whether her incontinence of the bowel and bladder that she has today is a permanent condition?

A. Yes, I think it's permanent.

Q. Will, in your opinion, Michelle require 24 care for the remainder of her days?

A. Yes.

Q. Do you foresee a time in the future where the amount of that care on a daily basis will diminish or will it remain at the 24-hour level?

A. I don't see it ever being less than 24 hours.

Q. Will Michelle require Ritalin for the rest of her life?

A. Yes.

Q. And why is that?

A. She has such extreme injury to her reticular activating system at the brain stem that she really needs external stimulation to stay aroused or awake. There may be some future medication that will be better than Ritalin, but I can't imagine that at least with the state of the present medical art that she would not require something to provide that.

Q. If Ritalin were discontinued today, would her arousal state diminish?

A. Yes.

Q. Would she return to a vegetative state?

A. Probably not all the way back to a vegetative state, but she's been unable to be consistently awake.

Q. In the future will in your opinion Michelle require any type of respiratory service?

A. She may well require help. She was a fairly weak cougher and should she get a respiratory illness, she would require chest BT and inhalation therapy. It is even conceivable that she would get sick enough that she would need to have a ventilator again, if she were to get a pneumonia, just because of her poor — the weakness of her muscles.

Q. What about future hospitalizations for Michelle, what do you envision in that regard?

A. Well, she certainly is at risk for infection. The big concern will be pulmonary and urine. The urine infections I would anticipate with good care could probably often be treated in the home. Because of her marginal pulmonary status, I think these infections will require hospital treatment.

These were just a few of the questions that were in the 138-page deposition. Where could I find hope after reading this? I had to pull up memories of Michelle to keep her intact. She seemed to be fading out of existence more and more and I wasn't going to let that happen. I thought of another saying on her wall: "You make more friends by becoming interested in other people than by trying to interest other people in yourself."

Michelle always attracted others to herself. And she did this not because she was trying to impress others but because she genuinely cared for them. Although her favorite group of individuals was children, she always had a large set of friends her own age and was also interested in the elderly. Frequently she'd drive her bike past Aunt Noreen's house and just stop in to say a quick hello. She would reach out to those individuals who had no friends and could see the goodness in them that others missed.

Because she was the youngest in a family of all boys, she grew up surrounded by men. Her best friend, Kara, also had three brothers, and they would often commiserate about what it was like to live with males. When she was in high school I remember she told me that she did not feel about boys the way her friends did. For her, there was nothing magical about them. She had seen first hand what they were capable of. She liked boys and always seemed to have a boyfriend, but she didn't need one to feel secure and did not go out of her way to attract them. She enjoyed going to an all girls' high school and filled her days with achievements rather than pursuit of boys.

In her senior year, she and a group of her friends were dating boys from Chaminade High School, a local all-boys school. Michelle's boyfriend, Dan, and some of his friends were all a year younger. This made a big difference because it meant that the girls had drivers' licenses and the boys did not. But this did not seem to bother anyone. The girls would pick the guys up, and they'd all go out together and have a great time. It did mean, however, that the girls would be driving home alone late at night. Michelle had a curfew and would always come charging into the driveway exactly at the time she was due home, not a minute earlier.

Similarly in college, Michelle was somewhat aloof about needing relationships with men, although she had many close male friends. They would confide in her, and she would help many through their romantic relationships. Because she was not a pursuer, males were very attracted to her. She had a deep appreciation of whom she was and did not need a man by her side to feel complete, although she did want to get married and have a family more than anything else in life.

In her senior year at the university, Michelle was a resident assistant and spent many hours talking and advising other students. It was a job she truly enjoyed, and she was wise beyond her years. Her concern for others and her ability to listen and be present were probably part of the reason she was attracted to psychology as a major. She would have been a good psychologist.

But I was never allowed to stay in the past too long. There were always decisions that needed to be made and roadblocks to negotiate. Although Michelle verbalized more, ate some pureed foods, spent some time on the tilt board to strengthen her bones, I could tell our days there were beginning to be numbered. She was not progressing sufficiently to justify her stay. One day when I arrived at Hartwyck, I noticed that Michelle's therapy schedule had been changed from three therapies every day to three therapies only three times a week. Eventually, I anticipated that the therapy schedule would be reduced further. I continued to research facilities on Long Island that would be able to provide Michelle with the level of therapy she needed.

In May, Dr. McCagg told me that Michelle would probably never be independent, but we still could not imagine what the future really held for Michelle. She was conscious, she knew who we were, and she knew she was loved and she told us that she loved us. But she was totally tube fed, was in diapers, drooled, and could not support her head without a headrest. It was still difficult for her to stay awake for extended periods, and cognitively she was still inconsistent with her responses. Her major deficit was her memory. Although she knew people and events from before the accident, she had little ability to maintain new information.

At the end of May, there was another family meeting, and we were told that therapy was again going to be dropped. Traveling to New Jersey every day had also begun to take its toll on us, so I decided to visit one of the few head injury units on Long Island, St. Johnland, in Kings Park. It was a fairly new facility attached to a nursing home. I toured the facility, spoke to the director, and after a phone call to Dr. Giacino at Hartwyck, I was told that Michelle would be admitted. The timing was right. Hartwyck was ready to get rid of us and St. Johnland had empty Medicaid beds on which they were losing revenue. I had learned the system well and always tried to stay one step ahead. Rather than wait for the social worker at Hartwyck to tell us that Michelle was going to be discharged I told her what our next stop would be. In two days Michelle would leave Hartwyck and be admitted to St. Johnland. Many arrangements needed to be made, but as always the family pulled together and did what was necessary. On June 10, 1999, Michelle left Hartwyck exactly one year after she entered the JFK-Johnson system. We will never forget the wonderful care and support we received there from everyone, especially Dr. McCagg. It was a tearful farewell, but it was time to move on.

7.

On June 10, 1999, when Michelle and I left Hartwyck, we traveled in a small ambulette with two drivers. Michelle was sitting in her wheelchair, strapped to the floor, and I sat beside her. Larry was in New Jersey loading her belongings into the car and would follow us to St. Johnland Head Injury Unit in Kings Park, Long Island. Several times during the trip to Long Island, Michelle screamed out in pain from the cramping in her leg, but most of the time she just sat there with her head bent slightly to the left and drooled. As I looked at her I couldn't help thinking of her as a little bird with a broken wing. I tried to imagine the future and what our lives would be like.

After close to two hours, we arrived at St. Johnland. Michelle was exhausted and was taken to her room, washed, and put to bed. I was relieved. We had arrived on Long Island, she was in a private room, and she would again have three hours of therapy every day. This would be a new beginning. I stayed with her the rest of the day and then went home, which now was only a half an hour away.

When I arrived the next day, Michelle seemed to be thriving. Perhaps the new surroundings had stimulated her. I took her outside in her wheelchair, and watched her as she did her therapies. Later I climbed into bed with her and watched a movie.

On Saturday evening I was in bed with her with my arm around her neck when I noticed something different. Her eyes looked funny. She seemed to be spaced out. She turned her head and just stared. It was just about time for me to leave but something seemed wrong, so I stayed a little longer. Then Michelle began to have a seizure. Although seizures are common after head injuries, she had never had one before. I rang for the nurse. When the nurse came, Michelle had another seizure. An ambulance was called, and we were to be taken to Stony Brook Hospital, which is a renowned teaching hospital on Long Island. The ambulance driver told us, however, that if anything happened on the way we would go to the closest hospital. Soon after we left, Michelle began to vomit. The driver made a turn, and we were taken to the closest hospital, which I knew did not have a good reputation.

We were rushed into the emergency room where Michelle was put on a table, examined by a nurse, and connected to a heart monitor. Soon afterwards, my son Tim, who lived close by, arrived. I had called my husband before we left St. Johnland, and he had notified our sons. Although Michelle seemed comfortable, she had not been given any medication. After about an hour, Michelle had another, more serious, seizure. She was hooked up to the heart monitor and I was amazed to see how hard her heart worked during the seizure. The doctor observed the seizure, gave her a dose of Dilantin, and then told me he wanted to admit her. I refused. I knew that if she were admitted to this hospital it would be difficult to get her out. I told him that we were on our way to Stony Brook Hospital and that we planned on continuing our trip. He reminded me that it was three o'clock in the morning. I told him that as far as I knew, hospitals did not close at night.

A short while later, an ambulance arrived and drove us to Stony Brook. When we arrived in the emergency room, the young doctor on duty wanted to tap Michelle's shunt to check for infection. I wouldn't allow him to do it. I had learned in Chicago that tapping Michelle's shunt was a last resort because it opened her to the possibility of infection. The doctor called a neurosurgeon who agreed with me.

Around one o'clock in the afternoon, Michelle was admitted to a room, and I stayed with her until my husband arrived. I was so tired; I needed to get some rest. Stony Brook was further away from our house than St. Johnland, and I could hardly drive home.

When I returned to the hospital on Monday, I found Michelle in her room, lying in bed covered in brown liquid. One of her medicines was brown, and when someone had fed her through her tube it must have backed up. Her hair, the wall behind her, and her bed were covered with specks of brown. I called the aide to wash Michelle.

Michelle was very unresponsive that day and the next but she had not had any more seizures. They determined that she had had a urinary track infection and that perhaps this was what caused the seizures.

Around 2:45 on Wednesday, an aide came and told me that Michelle had to be taken downstairs to the clinic to see the gynecologist. I asked why, and the aide said she didn't know and proceeded to put Michelle into a wheelchair. Michelle was so unresponsive, however, that she collapsed. Then the aide got a stretcher and loaded Michelle on it, while I kept asking why Michelle needed to see a gynecologist. I received no answer, so I followed the stretcher to the clinic. The aide reported in and told the staff members present to return Michelle to her room when they were finished. I told the aide not to leave until I knew why my daughter was here. I must have created quite a scene because the doctor came out and told me that when she saw Mrs. Burns that morning she wanted to follow up on something. I informed her that this was not Mrs. Burns. The aide had brought the wrong patient. So back we went to Michelle's hospital room. The aide dumped Michelle in bed and then got a wheelchair for Michelle's roommate. Her roommate was conscious, and the aide informed her that she was going downstairs to see the gynecologist, but the roommate responded that she was not Mrs. Burns. Mrs. Burns was two rooms down the hall. Again and again I learned the importance of always having an advocate by your side when you are in the hospital.

On Thursday, Michelle was released back to St. Johnland but she was very lethargic. The seizures and the medication seemed to have set her progress back tremendously. Just when I thought that she was getting better, there was a setback and we needed to start all over again. How would all of this end? It was like being on an emotional roller coaster ride, and all I could do was to keep going. There was no way to get off.

The summer passed this way. One day she would seem to make a little progress and then the next day she would be unresponsive. The hardest was on the weekends when there was no therapy, and I would arrive at St. Johnland only to find Michelle propped up in her wheelchair next to others in front of the nurses' station. She would be leaning to her left side and drooling. Sometimes I wasn't even sure if she knew that I was there. In addition, her bedroom had become infested with bees. There were bees flying around her room, but there was no empty room to which she could be transferred. They sprayed but I was also afraid of the fumes.

The head injury unit at St. Johnland was part of a nursing home, and to get to the coffee machine I had to walk through a part of the nursing home. As I saw all of the people lined up at the nurses' station I would always ask myself if they were like this solely because of their brain function, or did this environment contribute to their condition? I realized more and more how important environment is, and how our brains needed outside stimulation to function properly. The problem, of course, is that our current health-care system gives you few choices. If you do not make rapid progress in a rehabilitation facility you are sent to a nursing home, and then lack of recovery becomes the norm. Every place is short staffed, and people with brain injury need individualized attention. When you can't initiate on your own, others are needed to initiate for you.

I asked myself if I was putting too many demands on the system. Had the time come to accept that Michelle was not going to get any better? I thought of another quote from The Little Prince, "'Men' said the little prince, 'set out on their way in express trains, but they do not know what they are looking for. They rush about, and get excited, and turn round and round…'" Was that what I was doing? Again I turned to my professional training searching for answers.

I often said to Michelle when we had disagreements that she was more like a Taoist and I was more like a

Confucian. I was action oriented. It was hard for me to sit and do nothing, while she could spend hours just gazing at nature. I liked the city; she liked the country. Her accident had pulled me into her world. It had forced me to slow down, to sit and do nothing, to just wait. But on the other hand, I could not be complacent. Michelle's care depended on my being one step ahead of the professionals so I could assess the options that they offered me.

My favorite prayer has always been the serenity prayer because I think that it captures the true secret of life: "Lord grant me the serenity to accept the things I cannot change, the courage to change the things I can, and the wisdom to know the difference." Although Michelle had a better handle on acceptance than I, both acceptance and change are necessary to move things forward; the challenge is knowing when to do either.

My doctoral dissertation was on the virtue of prudence. There could not have been a better preparation for this ordeal. In fact, when my dissertation mentor, James Keenan, heard of Michelle's accident, he told me that I would do fine because I was comfortable with ambiguity, which is a recognized component in making prudent decisions. Many of the decisions I had to make about Michelle's care had no clear-cut answers. I needed to do damage control, make sure no further harm would come, or act without certainty that I was doing the right thing. Many times there was no prognosis, and I needed to function in the midst of doubt.

Prudence is the virtue that helps one make a decision in this situation. It asks the question, what is the most fitting thing to do here and now. It is personal. In other words, it is concerned with the concrete person in the present. For example, although there are general ethical guidelines about respirators and feeding tubes, prudence is needed to know if *now* is the time to withdraw a respirator or a feeding tube from this particular person. Prudence also considers that this is a twenty-one-year-old, otherwise healthy female, as opposed to an older person who is dying from a disease.

It takes circumstances as well as the person into consideration. Under our circumstances, I had determined that I would not put Michelle into a nursing home. If I had younger children, no husband, or no financial resources, I might have decided otherwise. As our circumstances change, so might Michelle's care plan.

Prudence requires looking forward, seeking possibilities for the future. This is probably where prudence helped me the most. I always tried to be one step ahead of the health-care professionals, so that when we had our family meetings, I would have some idea as to the options that would be in Michelle's best interest rather than in the best interests of a particular facility or the health-care system. As I look back, prudence helped me challenge so many of the decisions that I am sure would have had an adverse effect on Michelle's recovery: at Cook County Hospital, the staff had decided Michelle should go to the county rehabilitation facility, but I fought for her to be admitted to the Rehabilitation Institute of Chicago; at the Rehabilitation Institute, insurance dictated that Michelle be admitted to a nursing home on Long Island, but I fought for her to be admitted to JFK-Johnson; at JFK, staff again pushed to have Michelle discharged to a nursing home but I fought for her to be discharged to the subacute division of Hartwyck; at Hartwyck, when Michelle's therapy was reduced, I transferred her to St. Johnland. Without my foresight, few of these changes would have occurred. I accepted some things, like the seriousness of Michelle's injury but fought others, always focusing on getting her the best care possible. Many times, health-care professionals thought I pushed too hard and considered me to be irrational, but prudence is anything but complacent.

I also accepted Michelle's limitations and did not go to great lengths to try to eradicate these, but I continued to fight for all the standard therapy that Michelle needed in her recovery. It never made sense to me when professionals said that because Michelle was not improving, therapy should be decreased. It always seemed to me that if Michelle's response diminished she required either an increase in therapy or another type of therapy. I learned that with brain injury, you must never be complacent. The brain needs stimulation to grow, and if patients can't self-stimulate, others must do it for them.

On the other hand, I met many parents who attempted many different nontraditional therapies for their brain-injured children. I was not opposed to nontraditional means, as long as they would not harm Michelle. I ruled out hyperbaric treatment because I had heard of some individuals who had lung damage as a result of it. I would not go to India, as some did, to find herbs that might help her. I considered using gingko biloba to help with Michelle's memory, but rejected the idea when I was advised that it could also cause bleeding. But I did use a magnetic pillow, massage therapy, music, and exercise.

Prudence also demands that you learn from your experiences, and I was a quick learner. Before the accident, *rehab* was something I connected only with recovery from drug or alcohol dependency. I knew nothing about rehabilitation in Michelle's circumstances, but by having Michelle in one of the best rehabilitation facilities in the country, I was able to learn what good rehab comprises. I also learned how the health-care system works and what I needed to do to work the system. Some of the things I learned I had to draw on over and over again, and they became part of a checklist that I internalized:

- Never allow Michelle's shunt to be tapped, except as a last resort;
- Always make sure Michelle has an air mattress so that she doesn't develop bed sores;
- Keep Michelle's special boots on her at night so she doesn't get foot-drop;
- Do range of motion exercises with Michelle every day to avoid contractures;
- Follow Michelle everywhere, so transporters don't just drop her outside a room with no one to watch over her;
- Know Michelle's medications to avoid errors because her chart is so large that few physicians have time to read through it;
- Be pleasant to the nurses and aides because they're the ones who get you what you need and who watch over Michelle when you are not there;
- Track down therapists when they don't show up on time;
- Question physicians;
- Postpone family meetings as long as possible because they're always about discharge;
- Get to know someone in your insurance company so you have an insider fighting for you;
- Have an attorney subpoena something that you need when no one is responding to your request;
- Have a plan and compare it with the institution's plan, but remember the institution's staff ultimately must serve the institution rather than the patient;

- When it's time to move on to another facility, you may have to push hard enough to get into the facility of your choice that the staff at the current facility will be desperate to get rid of you and will help you to get into the next facility;
- Be Michelle's constant advocate and remember that no one knows her and what she needs as well as you do.

Prudence had served me well but prudence also told me that the time was soon coming when Michelle would be discharged. I also realized that all of my options were now used up. The system had saved Michelle's life but had few clues as to what to do with her now. The only thing left within the system was to put her into a nursing home. How does one put one's twenty-two year old daughter into a nursing home? Her friends were going to rock concerts and traveling throughout the world, and Michelle would be sitting with the elderly. I would never put Michelle in a nursing home. She would come home and live with us. I knew that this was the right thing to do, but I wasn't sure whether I was up to the task. Michelle was still totally tube fed, slept most of the day, and required twenty-four care. How would I care for her, go to work, and do the many other daily chores? But I had to try.

I thought of how Michelle did not pursue things so much as to prepare herself for them to come to her. Again a quote on her door captured this: "Happiness is a butterfly, which, when pursued, is always beyond your grasp. But which, if you will sit down quietly, may alight upon you." Usually they came. There were several times in high school when they did not. Michelle was not that active in sports but finally tried out for the badminton team, telling me that this was the team that everyone made who couldn't make any other sports team. She called me in the afternoon from school to say that she was a total sports failure. She hadn't made the team. Then she gave a little giggle and was ready to move on. She had tried, failed, and now it was time to move on to something else.

Much more devastating was the day she went for her driver's test and failed. But her friend Kara had failed also, and they turned it into a joke. They made fun of themselves, scheduled another appointment, and both passed the second time around. Michelle was disappointed but never let her disappointment consume her. Rather, she turned it into recognition of her humanity and moved forward. She never pretended to be perfect.

Perhaps most telling of how noncompetitive Michelle was happened at graduation from high school. Most of her friends were convinced that she would be valedictorian, but she was not. Instead Michelle had taken as many advanced placement courses as she could, rather than focus on the easier classes, which might earn her higher grades. She was not in the least upset that she came out third rather than first or second. For Michelle, it was not getting the prize that counted but how she performed along the way. Ironically, it was because she took these AP courses that she had enough credits to graduate from the University of Chicago at the time of her accident.

Michelle's greatest talents were in her writing. She was editor of her high school newspaper and wrote an editorial that earned her second prize from the Long Island newspaper, *Newsday*. The title was "Trust Me: A Critique of the 'SAFE (?) HOME' Program." It read as follows:

"Safe from drugs, safe from alcohol, safe from teenage parties." This is the slogan of the "SAFE HOME" program which has been adopted by Mercy in an attempt to "protect" us.

The "SAFE HOME" program asks parents to sign a pledge which states that they will not allow parties in their home when they are absent, nor will they allow drugs on their property. Those who sign the pledge are then listed as "safe parents" and every member of the program receives this catalog of names. This sounds like a great idea, the end to the threat of alcohol and forever! It is not.

In effect, the "SAFE HOME" program does not stop the problems of drugs and alcohol in our society; it cannot. The only success of this program is that it gives parents a false sense of security that their children are safe in an extremely unsafe world. Where is the real security in signing a piece of paper and having a list of names drawn up? These pieces of paper are not going to stop minors from drinking illegally, and they certainly are not going to stop an addict from obtaining drugs. The availability of these substances is too great; if the gang cannot drink at one house, they will find somewhere else to go.

Another problem with the "SAFE HOME" program is that is preaches against the normal growth process of a teenager. The ONLY way we will ever learn that we can say "No" is to be put in a situation where we will have to. Gold is tested in fire to determine its strength, yet we, according to the "SAFE HOME" program, must not be subjected to this pressured situation, lest we melt and be doomed forever. The biggest part of growing is learning how to avoid mistakes, or facing the consequences. During our teenage years when we are constantly pressured by outside influences, we cannot afford to have our decisions made for us. We have to discover for ourselves the basic truths which we need to lead a successful life.

Finally, what happens after high school? There does not exist a "SAFE COLLEGE" program." The argument that by then we will be mature enough to say no is a very weak one. It holds even less true if, throughout our high school years, we are completely guarded and conditioned to do exactly what our elders tell us. Being slapped in the face with total freedom after eighteen years of living under someone else's roof is not easy, in fact, it can be very harmful. That is why we must be trusted to taste freedom while we still have our parents to fall back on when we do the wrong thing.

There is only one way for parents to really protect their kids. It cannot be started in freshman year of high school, it must be started from day one. The only way children will ever grow up to be strong individuals is if they are shown strong values of self-respect, responsibility and trust from the very beginning. Once they develop these values, they must be rewarded with respect, responsibility, and trust from their elders, all the while being assured that they do have someone to fall back on when they mess up.

The "SAFE HOME" program tries to stunt this growing process by sending teenagers the message that there is an element of distrust. While this distrust may really be misinterpreted fear on the part of the parents, nothing is solved. Once again, a piece of paper is not going to change anything if the meaning behind it was not there in the first place. In fact, that piece of paper could actually make things worse when kids do interpret the fears and concerns of their parents as distrust.

The "SAFE HOME" program is an idealistic, abstract vision, one which can never be planted in reality. I am absolutely sure it was intended as a protective measure, established by concerned parents to help their children get through a tough age. However, it does not approach the real problem. Teenagers must grow up hearing themselves speaking in their own voices, not the voices of their parents. We must learn not only the decisions we should make, but also how and why we should come to certain conclusions. We need to learn to think for ourselves and face the consequences of our actions, not rely on others to think for us. Without these vital skills, developed mostly in teenage years, we can never advance to full adulthood of self-contentment.

This sounded like prudence at work to me. Maybe she was listening to me when I was working on my dissertation.

When Michelle went to college she was one of the founders and editors of *The Women's Guide to Health*. In addition to her editorial work, she contributed some of her drawings throughout the book. For example, heading the chapter on substance abuse, she drew a cigarette with the smoke coming out of it in the shape of a snake. The chapter on support groups had a sketch of someone walking on a tight rope with two women holding a safety net underneath. The book was comprehensive, covering everything from nutrition to substance abuse to women in cyberspace and much more. Each chapter also had a list of resources. I remember her spending the entire summer between her junior and senior year editing the guidebook.

And now we would be bringing this talented, intelligent, artistic, kind young woman home to live with us. But first I needed to do lots of preparations.

When I was still in Chicago, a physician had given me the name of a doctor on Long Island who specialized in brain injury. I had also heard of him when we were in New Jersey, so I knew that he was nationally known. I tracked him down and found him at Southside Hospital in Bayshore, Long Island. I called his office to see if he oversaw the care of TBI patients who lived at home. I thought that if I could find a doctor who could help me, maybe I could care for Michelle at home.

Dr. O'Dell's nurse told me that he did care for at-home patients, and I should make an appointment after we brought Michelle home. I got off the phone and thought about it for a moment, and then called her back saying that would not be sufficient. I wanted to see Dr. O'Dell for a consultation appointment now. She told me that insurance would not cover that, and I said that was fine, I'd do self-pay, but I needed to see the doctor.

In a few days, I went to see Dr. O'Dell. I liked him immediately. I told him a little about Michelle, and I stated that I did not think we still knew how much of her unresponsiveness was caused by her brain injury, and how much was caused by her drugs. I was convinced that she was over-drugged. He agreed with me but cautioned that there were risks involved with withdrawing some drugs. I understood but told him that we would never know how far Michelle could progress unless we took those risks.

Together we decided that the best way to test the drug protocol was to do drug withdrawal in a hospital setting. We would put Michelle in Southside Hospital for a few weeks before we brought her home. Dr. O'Dell would get to know her and then oversee her care when she was home. He told me he would have to check with administration if this could be done because it had never been done before, but I reminded him that there was a discharge plan in place so there should not be a problem. I had learned the system well.

While Michelle was still at St. Johnland, she was evaluated for nursing services. It was agreed that she could receive sixteen hours of licensed practical nurse (LPN) services when she came home. Medicaid would pay for that. We also found an agency that would provide those services.

At the beginning of October, Larry and I picked up Michelle at St. Johnland and took her to Southside Hospital. She was examined, put into a room, and slowly weaned from some of her drugs. The goal was to withdraw the Dilantin and replace it with Neurontin. We were also withdrawing Ritalin, which had been used to help stimulate her. She also received therapy and underwent another swallow test to be sure that we could again begin to feed her by mouth. At St. Johnland, the staff fed her only through her tube.

We were back in another institutional, bureaucratic setting. The weekend after we had admitted Michelle, I asked if I could take her outside for a walk. I was told I could not because I had not yet had wheelchair training. I had been pushing her in a wheelchair for close to two years, had brought her to the hospital in her wheelchair, but I was under hospital rules again. I told the staff to give me wheelchair training, but the person who did that was off for the weekend, so Michelle and I could not leave the floor of the hospital. I couldn't wait to get her home and be in charge.

Our daily routine continued. I went to work, and my sons and my husband each continued to spend one day a week with Michelle. I would call every day that I was not there to keep updated on what was happening. One evening when the aide came in to take Michelle for her shower, I noticed that she was very unresponsive. I asked the aide to check Michelle's oxygen level, which she did and told me that it was seventy-two. I told her to call the doctor right away that Michelle was in danger. The nurse came running into the room and, it turned out that the aide had mistaken her pulse number for her oxygen number. Nevertheless, the physician on call came because Michelle was extremely unresponsive. She was slipping back into unconsciousness. The following day her Ritalin was restarted, and she again became more alert.

The time was fast approaching when Michelle would come home. We were making arrangements at home. Our den, in the front of our house, was converted to her bedroom. It was small but adequate. We moved her supplies into the closet, bought a hospital bed, put in a rocking chair for the nurses and waited for Michelle's arrival. Although we would be provided with LPNs for sixteen hours a day, I knew I needed nurses around the clock. I recognized my limitations and knew that this would be my life now for a long, long time. I needed to make this as easy as possible if it was going to work, and it had to work because there was no way I could put my daughter into a nursing home. I just wasn't sure how I would do this.

I had found a speech therapist who would work with Michelle when she came home. She lived in Rockville Centre, which was about half an hour from our home. I also spoke to some of the therapists at the hospital and an occupational therapist (OT) and physical therapist (PT) agreed to come to our home to work with Michelle. In addition, someone had told me about a therapy called feldenkrais, which deals with movement and balance and would help Michelle relearn her body. This therapist practiced one day a week in Great Neck, so we would take Michelle to him.

I asked, Lisa, who had taken care of Michelle when we brought her home on weekends if she would be interested in working more regularly for us. She agreed to work two days a week for us. Then the mother of one of Michelle's friends, Laura, happened to mention to me that she was looking for a job. I asked her if she would be interested in working with Michelle. Laura had gone to New Jersey to see Michelle one day a week for a long time, so I knew that she loved her. She had no credentials, but neither did I, and I knew that Laura would be great. I was so excited when she agreed to work two days. Then I found Kinga, who would do one day. I would use these people for the day shifts and the agency nurses for the evening and night shifts. For the time being, I would be the nurse on Saturdays and Sundays.

Everything seemed to be falling into place, and then, two days before Michelle was to come home, the agency that was supposed to take our case informed the hospital that it could not find nurses to staff the case. Medicaid pays lower wages than insurance cases, so nurses want to work on insurance cases and not on Medicaid cases. The hospital was searching frantically for another agency because Michelle could not be released until a plan was in place, and it was time for her to leave the hospital.

Finally, the hospital found an agency that could provide the required nurses. I had never heard of this agency, and called Albany, our state capital, to make sure that agency was registered. The agency was registered, but it was very small. I accepted the agency's services, signed the necessary papers, and on Tuesday, November 3, 1999, we picked up Michelle at the hospital and brought her home. After almost two years in hospitals and rehabilitation facilities, Michelle would be coming home to live with us, and I would be responsible for her care. It was an awesome and frightening responsibility. Again I wondered whether I would be up to the task. But by the time we left Southside Hospital, I knew a great deal about rehabilitation. I could also tell who was a good nurse or a good therapist within about five minutes. The good ones, I found, viewed their jobs as a vocation and not just as a paycheck. I found that as time passed and as we moved further and further away from acute care facilities the balance of knowledge and power began to tilt away from the professionals and move in my direction.

I had also learned over and over again the need for community. I could not have learned all that I did by reading books, although books offered me great consolation. I needed to see others in action. I needed to see good therapists and bad; good doctors and bad; good nurses and bad; good aides and bad in order to learn the differences. Sometimes the differences are so subtle (a tone of voice, the speed with which someone does something), that you always must be alert and present. I respected most those professionals who were honest, did not patronize me, and recognized me as an important part of Michelle's care. Medicine is an art as much as a science, and the best professionals know this. What I did not realize right away, but what I know now, is that I also needed time to learn all of this. Now that I was bringing Michelle home, it was important that I had had time in rehabilitation facilities to learn what I needed to know to properly care for her and to develop the appropriate skills. I had come to know some of the best professionals in the field, and now I needed to take what I had learned and put it into action. I hoped that prudence would again serve me well to face the new challenges of caring for Michelle at home. Home would be the place where my professional and personal knowledge would coalesce and where we would help Michelle forge her new identity.

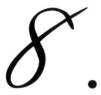

8.

At Home

_____

On the way home from the hospital, we stopped at a hospital supply factory to have Michelle's wheelchair adjusted. She would be spending a great deal of time in her chair, and having a proper fit was extremely important. Just sitting in a wheelchair required a tremendous amount of energy for Michelle.

Soon after we arrived home and after I had changed Michelle, did the tube feeding, and placed her in bed, the agency nurse came to do the necessary paperwork. The first nurse from the agency was to arrive at 11pm that evening, and the paperwork needed to be completed before that. I had to sign many forms, which established our relationship with the agency. The one most clear in my memory was a DNR (do not resuscitate) order. I refused to sign that. Michelle was severely brain injured but she was not dying. She required a great deal of care, but it was basic care like feeding, bathing, turning in bed, and stretching. So frequently health-care professionals viewed this kind of care as burdensome, while respirators, transplants, and brain surgeries had become run of the mill. Advanced technology and medical skill and expertise saved Michelle's life at age twenty-one, but it would take more basic equipment and skills to care for Michelle for the rest of her life, and the health-care system seemed ill-prepared to provide quality long-term care for Michelle over the long haul.

When the paperwork was completed, the nurse left; I waited for the night nurse to arrive, but she did not. I kept calling the agency, and, finally, around 1am I was informed that no nurse was available. I had to go to work the next morning. My son Nick came and stayed downstairs with Michelle while I went up to bed. He turned her every two hours, which was necessary so she would not get bed sores, and woke me if she needed to have her diaper changed or if it was time to give her medicines. We made it through the night, and Laura arrived at 7am to begin her first day of work with Michelle. Laura had gone for training at Southside Hospital and had learned how to do the feedings, give the medicines, do the transfers, etc. Michelle had not had any seizures since that June night in St. Johnland, but we were still not sure whether she would have another. I left for work and left Laura in charge, but I called home between each of my classes to make sure that all was going well. Fortunately, my husband worked close by should any emergency develop, and I was only thirty-five minutes away.

I was now in charge but I began to feel like I wasn't going to get much help. There were so many details to take care of and no central place to go for resources. Our future depended on me figuring out how to put a plan together and then how to execute it. Larry and the boys had been with me every step of the way but now that we were home it was more or less assumed that because I was the mother I should do what I have always done – take care of my child. But my daughter had left as an independent, competent young woman and she was returning requiring twenty-four hour care. Cooking and laundry were now added to the daily chores. I also had my teaching career and my tenure date was only a year away. I had to publish. How was I going to do this? I resolved I would do what I had done since the day of the accident. I would take one day at a time. It was impossible to plan a future. None of us knew how things would turn out. Michelle had survived and I had promised her I would stand by her. I don't break promises.

We got through the first day. Everything went smoothly for Laura and Michelle. The agency nurse arrived at 3pm. She was a young woman named Marlo, an LPN, and she had another young woman with her whom she was training. Marlo worked well with Michelle and had an infectious laugh that lightened up the atmosphere and calmed Michelle. The young trainee, however, had just given birth and spent a great deal of time in the bathroom pumping her milk and missing her newborn. At 11pm, the night nurse arrived, and Marlo and I went over the routine with her.

Thus began what would be a daily routine for us – days filled with what Marion Deutsche Cohen calls in her book, *Dirty Details* (Temple University Press, 1996). These are the repetitive chores that are basic but low-skilled – chores that no one gives much thought to unless there is no one there to do them. We were now entering the world of long-term care and beginning to encounter the many frustrations that came with that world. I also found it strange that people stopped visiting. Individuals who came faithfully to the facilities didn't come to the home. Did they feel like they were intruding? Were they ready to move on? Where was I going to find my new source of strength? Part of the issue could have been my fault as well. Now that we were home I didn't have time to sit and entertain guests. Nevertheless, I felt like people were beginning to forget Michelle. That was the hardest thing for me to accept. I began to resent those who left us and it hurt most when those who had been faithful the longest left because then there was no one. Yet, as I thought about it more, they may have thought that now that we were home things had normalized. We, however, were not yet sure what normal meant.

There were nurses in and out of our house twenty-four hours a day and we had no privacy. I was glad our home had two stories. Upstairs was still a little private and the upstairs bathroom became my sanctuary. It was the only place I could be alone. So many people had told me to be careful of strangers in my home. But they were only strangers if I treated them as strangers. I welcomed them. I was extremely grateful to have others help me care for my daughter. I did not think of them so much as employees as assistants, for I knew that I could not do this on my own. How fortunate I was to have others who were qualified to help me care for Michelle. And, after what we had been through already, I had little concern about things being stolen, although I did hide the silverware.

Some of the nurses, worked only a few shifts and then dropped out, but eventually we had a reliable team in place. The people we had hired, Laura, Lisa, and Kinga, covered the 7am to 3pm shift, Darlene and Marlo covered the 3pm to 11 pm shift, and Guylourdes and Glory covered the 11pm to 7am shift. These were all hard-working and dedicated individuals who gradually became integrated into our family. All came to love Michelle. This was the new social circle we were beginning. I hadn't planned on having so many different nurses. This is just how things fell into place. But as I thought about it, it was a great plan. For many of these women this was their second job so they could cover for each other if needed.

I also started Michelle on scheduled therapies. The physical therapist, John, came to the house twice a week. He mainly stretched Michelle and gave electric stimulation to try to activate some of her muscles. Tami, an occupational therapist, arrived twice a week. Once a week we took Michelle to her speech therapist, Dr. Carol Manly, in Rockville Centre. At Michelle's first visit, Dr. Manly put a letter board in front of Michelle thinking she might use that to communicate. Michelle pushed it away, she wanted to talk; not point to letters. She also began feldenkrais with Dr. Ofir, who had Michelle lie on a table to help her relearn her body; for example by having her pass her fingers over her lips.

At home, the nurses worked very diligently on helping Michelle relearn how to eat. Eating is a very difficult task. To begin with, Michelle needed to be in a room alone with a nurse. There could be no distractions. All of Michelle's limited energy needed to be focused on the task at hand. After every small mouthful, the nurse would have to remind Michelle to chew and swallow. She would forget that she had food in her mouth. The first foods Michelle ate were soft foods like bananas, yogurt, and pureed foods. Even these foods caused her problems, and she would sometimes gag and cough before she swallowed. But we were persistent. In the beginning, it would take about an hour to have Michelle eat four ounces of applesauce. She was still tube fed but we supplemented that with mouth feedings, hoping to eventually remove the feeding tube. Over time we progressed to more textured food. Saturday mornings, I would usually spend two hours with Michelle feeding her one slice of French toast. We eventually cut her tube feedings back and added more solid food as well as protein drinks. The last things that were added to her diet were thin liquids, water, and juices. Thin liquids go down the throat very quickly, and there was a risk that Michelle would aspirate them into her lungs. We needed to be very careful with them.

When Michelle came home from Southside Hospital, she was taking 100 mg of Dilantin, 2700 mg of Neurontin, and 40 mg of Ritalin. Our goal was to get her off the Dilantin entirely and eventually wean her from the Ritalin and Neurontin. Because she was at home, we were able to do this much more slowly than in the hospital, where we needed to have quick results. The first medication to go was the Dilantin. Once she was off the Dilantin, she became much more responsive. Now she was able to complete her hour of therapy, whereas, when she was in rehabilitation facilities, she often fell asleep in the middle of therapy. After an EEG, which detected that there was no seizure activity present, and under the guidance of Dr. O'Dell, we also began to wean her from the Neurontin, but this was over a period of months. We likewise decreased the Ritalin. There was no question that drugs were a necessary part of Michelle's care, but they had to be carefully monitored because they could also produce adverse side effects and counteract the benefits of other drugs.

Sometime in the beginning of 2000, I began to overhear my agency nurses complaining to each other. Evidently, some of the checks that the agency had given to the nurses had insufficient funds to back them. I knew that if this continued I would lose my nurses. Who would want to work under these conditions? I approached them and asked them if they would be willing to continue working with Michelle if I transferred the case to a more reputable agency. They all wanted to continue with Michelle, but they also needed to get paid. I called the agency with which we had originally intended to contract; that agency could not take our case because it did not have nurses. When I approached the agency about taking the case and having my nurses transfer to the agency, the agency agreed to take the case. The agency had the benefit of getting a case already set up, and all it had to do was to process the paperwork and collect the profit. Generally, leaving an agency and taking the nurses on the case with you to another agency is not permitted; however, because the original agency had written so many bad checks, I knew that it would be difficult for them to fight me. The agency was small, and, as I found out later, Michelle's case was the agency's first Medicaid case, and so there was a delay in payment. The agency found that it could not cover payments to the nurses until the Medicaid payment arrived.

There was a transitional period where it was difficult. In fact, for several weeks, we paid the nurses with our own funds, but eventually everything was in place and the new agency administered the case and the nurses were again getting regular payments from an agency.

There were many days when I felt like an automaton. Sitting back and reflecting on what had happened or pausing and allowing my emotions to come front and center were luxuries I did not have. Since the accident food became my source of comfort. Other mothers in these facilities smoked and drank coffee while I ate. I knew I had gained a great deal of weight but that too would need to be put on the back burner. There really was no time to think of myself, and Larry and the boys were pretty much on their own. But Michelle continued to make progress and became more alert. She improved in therapy, and the therapists had also given us practice exercises to do with Michelle between therapies. Finding therapists to work in the home is difficult, however. There is no central location to go to where you can hire therapists. I found a cognitive therapist through an agency, but the therapist was young and inexperienced and would simply play music for Michelle and take her for walks. I felt that we could do this ourselves, so after a short period of time I let him go. The individual therapists who worked with Michelle often did not arrive as scheduled. They worked all day in the hospital, and viewed working with Michelle as less of a priority–it earned them extra money but if they were tired or had other things to do they would cancel their appointments with Michelle. I decided that I had to have as many nurses and therapists as possible working with Michelle so that I would be assured of some therapy for her even if some therapist did not show up. I also found that this allowed Michelle to benefit from the widest range of skills: some therapists and nurses were excellent at grooming, some were more patient and did the tedious things better, some were more fun, some were better at the physical aspects of therapy, some at the cognitive, some introduced her to music, some to silence. Diversity was the key. No one provided everything, but together we had developed a good care plan.

I was always on the lookout for good therapists and nurses. I never relied on the agency to supply them for me. Because we had brought our nurses to the agency and never used any agency nurses, I felt we were in control of the case. If someone could not work, we arranged a substitute among ourselves. We never called the agency for a replacement. Everything focused on Michelle.

In a short period of time, our occupational therapist left. She had been traveling a great distance, and it became too difficult for her to come. I found a company that provided OT in the home that was run by a husband and wife team. The husband was a neuropsychologist and the wife was an occupational therapist. The day that the neuropsychologist came to do his evaluation was the same day that the nurse from Medicaid came to do her evaluation. They both arrived at the same time. In order to continue nursing services and not be downgraded to aides, Michelle needed to appear to be making little progress. Nursing services were required to do tube feedings, and although Michelle still was tube fed, we did not want the evaluator to know how much Michelle was eating on her own. On the other hand, to get cognitive services, Michelle needed to show that she was making sufficient progress. So in one room Michelle needed to appear in bad condition, and in another she needed to shine. Laura was the nurse that day and had a hard time remembering if she was in the slow room or the fast room.

As Michelle began to eat more by mouth, we also began to experience some problems with her feeding tube. Sometimes it was drawn into her stomach. There were other times when it fell out. I knew that if the tube fell out that it needed to be replaced as quickly as possible so that the opening would not close. The first time this happened, I rushed Michelle to the local hospital, which did not have a G-tube the size Michelle needed so the staff inserted a catheter into her stomach. I wasn't satisfied with this solution. Fortunately, a friend's son sold hospital supplies, and he was able to deliver three

G-tubes to my house that were the proper size. Several days later, the catheter fell out, and I had to take Michelle back to the hospital. But now I had the proper tube, which I took with me and had the hospital staff insert. When Michelle was in institutions, we as family were restricted from doing anything. We were treated as incompetent and our opinions were never solicited. Now that Michelle was home I even needed to find my own medical supplies. I was discovering that institutions were only concerned about what you did while the patient was under their jurisdiction. For example, when the agency nurses were on duty everything had to be documented. When they left nothing was documented. I understood the reasoning but it also made me feel like they really didn't care about Michelle but only that nothing adverse would happen while they could be held accountable. They wanted to protect themselves more than care for Michelle.

Around this time, Michelle's physical therapist, John, told me that he was moving to Florida. This meant that I would need to find a new physical therapist. We still had Dr. Manly, working with Michelle's speech; Dr. Ofir doing feldenkrais; and Rita doing occupational therapy as well as her husband giving cognitive services. But we needed a new physical therapist. Dr. Ofir came to the rescue. He had a friend who ran a physical therapy facility, and a young physical therapist there specialized in brain injuries. We called Christine, and she agreed to work with Michelle. She began to come to the house two days a week.

In May, when my semester of teaching was over, I also decided to have my knees replaced. I could barely walk anymore, and was in constant pain. I had put the surgery off because Michelle required all our attention, but I couldn't wait any longer. I was going to have both my knees done at the same time because I didn't have time to go through this twice. I found a doctor at the Hospital for Special Surgery in New York City and scheduled the procedure. I had nurses in the house for Michelle, and I knew that they would help me if I needed them. After several weeks of doing the prep work, Larry drove me to the hospital, and I underwent surgery. I asked my friend Lisa, who lived close to the hospital, to become my health-care proxy, because I wanted Larry to focus on Michelle. Lisa stayed with me every day and watched over me. After five days, I was discharged and came back to Long Island to North Shore Hospital at Glen Cove for rehabilitation. I had worked very hard exercising my knees before the surgery, and it paid off now. My first day in rehabilitation, the therapist gave me a cane with which to walk. I worked diligently, because I knew I had to get home to Michelle, and after a week I was discharged. The day I returned home I was able to walk up the stairs to my bedroom. I had a rapid recovery, although I was very tired for most of the summer.

During Michelle's first six months at home, we had succeeded in reducing her medication (she was now completely off the Dilantin, and we were also able to reduce the Neurontin and Ritalin), and taught her to eat by mouth. We were also able to strengthen her neck muscles, increase her lung capacity so she could say several words, improve her standing transfers from bed to wheelchair, and increase her alertness. Finally, on July 7, her feeding tube was removed. She had been fed by the tube for over two years.

That summer we also began to plan an addition to the back of our house. Michelle had been in a little room in the front of the house since she returned home. She spent most of her time in that room or the living room with us. She had had only bed baths. We wanted her to have a room of her own with lots of light, a bathroom where she could have showers, and a therapy area where we could put equipment. We had an architect draw up the plans, and we hired our neighbor Jake and his brother, Bruce, who are builders, to begin work on an extension to our home that could accommodate Michelle's new life style. I wanted lots of light in her room because I wasn't sure how much time Michelle would be spending in her bed, and I wanted her to be able to look at the trees and flowers from her bed. Construction work began in the fall and continued until the next spring. During this time, nurses and therapists worked in the front of the house with Michelle while the construction crew worked at the back of the house.

Rita helped us pick out equipment for Michelle's therapy area. We ordered a fold-down mat on which she could do physical therapy, a standing frame (a large box with knee supports and back supports) in which she could stand upright everyday, and a shower chair, which would fit over the toilet and in which she could get her shower. Once the addition was complete we also planned to begin toilet training.

Because Michelle had little movement on the right side of her body, I instructed the staff to do everything for Michelle from the right side. She was right handed, and I knew how confusing it would be if she now needed to learn how to do things with her left hand. In addition, although her right side was much weaker than her left side, she did not have as much ataxia (shaking) in her right hand, so she had better control. Everything I read about the brain reinforced "use it or lose it" theory. That became our motto. I was convinced that if Michelle was going to make any progress, it would be because we forced her to repeat certain functions over and over again. We could not give up. We would use her body to retrain her mind. She was home. We now had the time to do it. I also recognized that as some of the lower-function activities, such as chewing, became more automatic, she had more energy to give to the higher function activities.

Most of what we were doing was experimental. The therapists were there to guide us, but none of us knew how Michelle would respond to any of this. We could only take each day at a time and not get discouraged when there was very slow progress or no progress. We loved Michelle regardless of what condition she was in, and I found it impossible to set goals. I had no delusions that she would soon become independent, but I also would not abandon my daughter or not help her to become all she could be.

As Michelle continued to work and begin to form her new identity I thought of the work of William James, a famous psychologist, and how he used the concept of a stream of consciousness to describe the unbroken flow of consciousness that creates the core or essence of an individual and that remains even as events and experiences continue to change the individual. According to James' construct, it's as though we have two selves: the permanent self and the ever-changing self.

For someone like Michelle who has suffered a severe brain injury, it is as though the stream of consciousness has gone over a waterfall. The essence of who Michelle is remains, and yet, due to a traumatic event, that part of her identity that changes has not done so gently but has suffered through the violent turbulence at the bottom of the waterfall–crashing and fracturing but still remaining, just as the rushing water at the bottom of the waterfall gathers itself up and maintains its direction. There are so many pieces that now need to be put back together.

The neurologist Antonio Damasio refers to core consciousness and extended consciousness. Core consciousness is that part of one's self that stays the same; extended consciousness, on the other hand, is what connects the lived past to the anticipated future. It was obvious that Michelle still maintained her core consciousness. She knew who she was. She knew all of us whom she had known pre-accident. Soon after she emerged from the coma, she was even able to tell her therapists her home phone number. She knew all the information she had known prior to the accident. What was missing was her ability to integrate the person she had become and the events that occurred around her on a daily basis into her core identity.

For example, she would tell us that she could walk. Yet, every time she would try to stand she would lose her balance. She clearly remembered walking more than she remembered losing her balance, even though she may have lost her balance only a minute before.

She constantly spoke of getting married and having children. This is what she had wanted before her accident and saw no reason why that would not still happen. When we used this information to try to motivate her to stop repeating over and over again her desire for diapers, she informed us that her husband would understand. If he did not, she wouldn't marry him. Part of this was the old Michelle, not ashamed of whom she was, while at the same time not having any recognition that diapers may not be appealing to a new husband.

It was also around this time that the lawsuit was settled in Chicago, but before the Chicago courts would release the money, Larry and I had to go to court on Long

Island to be appointed Michelle's guardians. I had already been in court in Chicago and appointed her guardian, but I had to go through the process again in New York. Two attorneys from the family court system came to our home to interview us and to inspect our care of Michelle. Our sons also needed to be interviewed. This was so difficult. We had been by our daughter's side constantly for three years, and now two strangers entered our home and had the power to recommend that our daughter be taken away from us. Although I understood why this protocol is required, I still could not help but feel angry and humiliated that strangers were passing judgment on my relationship with my daughter.

The attorneys were considerate, and in several weeks we went to court. The judge listened to the attorneys' report and then listened to our testimony as to what had happened to Michelle and how we planned to care for her. Michelle was with us and also testified. We were appointed her legal guardians and then sent to classes to learn how to do all the necessary reporting and paper work involved in guardianship. And there is a great deal to do. A judge was appointed to oversee Michelle's care, and every spring we must submit a detailed report to him that documents every doctor's appointment Michelle has had, every hour of therapy, every change in medication, every social activity in which she has participated. We also need to justify where we have spent every penny of her money. In addition to this, we needed to take out a bond to cover her estate in case we absconded with her funds. Fortunately, Larry is very adept at computers and records all the necessary information electronically so that the twenty-page annual report becomes manageable. Often, we have been asked to further clarify something that we submitted on the report.

When we were at court, the judge also stated that Michelle had suffered a great deal, and he expected to see in our yearly report that we had taken her on a vacation. So we began to plan a spring vacation for her. As we did our research, we learned that it is convenient to take persons in wheelchairs on cruises. You must plan these trips far in advance, however, because the handicapped-accessible rooms on cruise ships are limited. In addition, because the staterooms and bathrooms are larger than in other areas of the ship, a doctor's note is also required that states that an individual actually has a disability because many people who do not have a disability try to obtain these rooms.

After some research, we decided to take a May cruise to Bermuda. The ship was sailing out of New York, so it would be much easier than first flying with Michelle to another destination. We also decided that we would turn this into a family vacation. Our sons had played a major role in Michelle's recovery, and none of us had had a break in three years, so in May of 2001 we all went to Bermuda. Two of Michelle's nurses, Darleen and Glory, agreed to accompany us.

Several weeks before the cruise, I went for my annual mammogram and discovered that I had breast cancer. I dealt with it very matter of factly as I did with everything but I was angry, very angry. Larry and I were about to enter "our golden years." In fact, many of our friends had already retired and were traveling, playing golf, and enjoying themselves. I didn't mind missing out on that. All I wanted to do was to care for my daughter. It was impossible for me to get sick or die. My daughter needed me. Surely, God could understand that. I was scheduled to have a lumpectomy ten days before we were to sail for Bermuda. This trip was important. Our entire family was going to go, and it was the first time that we would be taking Michelle away. I decided to have the surgery, go on the trip, and then begin treatment when I returned. The surgery went well. It was outpatient surgery, and I was home by 4:30 the same day.

There was another glitch to our travel plans: The day before we were to leave, Michelle had a doctor's appointment, and Dr. O'Dell thought that she might have a blood clot in her leg. We were able to get an appointment that same day for a Doppler test. Fortunately, she did not have a blood clot, and we finished packing our bags and took off for Bermuda. It turned out to be a wonderful but exhausting trip. While in Bermuda we also had Michelle swim with the dolphins. We put her in a wetsuit, and with her brothers she sat in the water and played with the dolphins.

When we came home I met with my oncologist and was told that I did not need chemotherapy only radiation treatment. I was thrilled. When I met with the radiologist he explained the procedure to me and ended by saying that he knew that he had given me a great deal of information and that I was probably emotionally distraught. I told him to stop right there. Then I told him a little about Michelle and ended by saying that for me this cancer was a nuisance. It was something that needed to be taken care of. I was taking care of it now it was time to move on. Everything seemed minor compared to the ordeal we had gone through with Michelle. I hated when people patronized me.

When Michelle was in rehabilitation facilities, we were told that she had had damage to her frontal lobes, which control executive functions of her brain, and that she would probably never be able to initiate conversation, set goals, etc. In other words, when we asked

Michelle a question she responded appropriately, but she did not ask us questions. Her major deficit also was her short-term memory. She could remember the things she knew before the accident, but she had a hard time remembering new facts and faces. Every day a nurse who had been working with her for over a year would have to reintroduce herself, but people she knew in grade school, she still remembered. We were told that she would probably be like this the rest of her life.

In trying to find new ways to improve Michelle's memory, I decided to try to draw on her academic work at the University of Chicago, where she was a psychology major. I contacted my colleagues at St. John's University and asked whether Michelle could audit a psychology class. I carefully chose the professor, and, in September, Michelle began to go to Saint John's two days a week and, with her nurse, sat in on an abnormal psychology class. She had already had the course at the University of Chicago, and I was hoping that it would spark some memories. By the end of the semester, she began to raise her hand and ask questions. She was initiating.

Michelle's physical therapist, Christine, told us about a special skiing program for persons with disabilities conducted in upstate New York at Windham Mountain. There were chair-skis there and trained volunteers who helped persons with disabilities ski down the mountain. We scheduled a weekend of skiing. Michelle met the qualifications. She was finally able to hold her head up without a headrest. This was important for skiing down the mountain.

Christine and some of her friends, two of our sons, my daughter-in-law Melissa, Larry and I, and Michelle went to Windham for a weekend of skiing. It was quite an entourage. Everyone, except Larry and I, went up on the chairlift with Michelle and together skied down. In addition to our group, who cheered Michelle on, there were three trained volunteers. One held the ropes that guided the chair-ski, and two skied beside her. What Michelle needed to do was to shift her weight in the chair in order to direct it. It was an exhilarating day.

I did not have a nurse with me that weekend, so I took care of Michelle when we went back to the hotel room. That evening she stayed awake most of the night insisting that she had to go to the bathroom, yet when I took her, she would not relieve herself. This occurred at least five or six times and was exhausting. We had been toilet training Michelle for the past several months, and it was quite an ordeal. In the beginning, we would place Michelle's shower chair over the toilet seat because she needed the support of a headrest and arm rests. Now, however, she could sit right on the toilet, but sometimes she would sit there for long periods of time.

I mark this night as the beginning of what I came to later call, "the year from hell." Once Michelle was off all her medicine, the temper tantrums began. I had seen this bad behavior in the rehabilitation facilities, but I had thought that because Michelle had been unconscious for such a long period of time that she had missed this stage, but now I was wrong.

We never knew what would trigger a tantrum. The slightest provocation, such as someone knocking at the door, could set her off. She would begin to scream, curse, and kick. It was getting impossible to take her out in public. My daughter, who had never cursed in her life, now came out with strings of curses. And she usually said them quite loudly.

I struggled for a long time trying to decide how to handle this. I did not want to drug Michelle just to control her, but on the other hand if we did not do something we were going to lose our staff. In addition, Michelle's social life was becoming more limited because of her behavior. It was so providential that we had such a large staff because it was becoming more and more difficult to work with Michelle.

We tried working with behavioral specialists, and Dr. O'Dell worked with me trying to find a medication that might help Michelle gain a little more control. There was one weekend when we started her on the drug Provigil. She began to hallucinate and did not sleep for four days. We quickly weaned her from that drug.

I had received tenure the year before and took a sabbatical the fall semester of 2002. We planned a family vacation to Disney World for December. Glory, our nurse, was coming with us. Disney World is a wonderful place to go with someone who is in a wheelchair. Everything is handicapped-accessible, and it is not necessary to wait in line. We chose a hotel that was on the grounds so we could easily roll Michelle right on to the monorail. We drugged her to get her on the plane so she would not scream and kick during the flight and hoped for the best when we arrived at Disney World.

It was a pleasant trip, although Michelle's behavior was very bad at times. Her attention span was short, so as soon as something ended, such as a ride or dinner, she was not able to just sit and wait. She needed to go on to the next activity or she would begin to kick and scream. It was like watching the behavior of a two-year-old. At one point, she even kicked a sliding door off its grid.

This behavior was also affecting her therapies. If she did not want to do a therapy, and it was usually physical therapy, she would begin to act up. Add this to her short-term memory issues, where she could not remember that she had just eaten or just gone to the bathroom, and life was becoming unbearable. We all struggled, never quite sure if this behavior was due to her brain injury or whether she was doing it to manipulate us. We suspected that it was a combination of both and wondered how long it could go on. Although she continued to make some progress, especially in speech therapy, it was hard to get beyond the bad behavior. I was so grateful for the days that I went to work and thankful that I had a devoted staff that did not leave us.

Around this time it was also recommended to us that we put Michelle into a day program for head injured persons. This was to help with her socialization. These were structured days where Michelle would be part of a group and do cognitive exercises as well as receive occupational therapy. These programs were very expensive, however, so to do this we had to apply for the Medicaid waiver. This is a program that New York State has to help individuals with disabilities who live at home. It finances several activities so that these persons may continue to live with their families rather than be placed in an institutional setting. To obtain these services, Medicaid recipients must go through a lengthy application process. The program also requires that the disabled individual have a case manager, someone who directs the individual and looks after his or her well-being.

I was very intent on finding an independent case manager. Many who are qualified to be case managers also work in established programs. For example, the social worker at the day program in which we hoped to have Michelle accepted, Transitions of Long Island, was a certified case manager. I had been in the system long enough, however, to know that someone who worked at an institution was likely to direct the client to their institution. I wanted someone whose primary concern was Michelle and who would direct her to wherever was best for her. We were very fortunate to find Barbara, a New York State certified independent case manager who worked extremely well with us.

We were successful in obtaining the Medicaid waiver and enrolled Michelle in the program at Transitions, which she attended two days a week. An aide went with her to help her with lunch and toileting. The tantrums continued but she was in brain injury units with qualified staff. For these few hours I felt like she was their problem. They're trained to deal with this type of patient. I finally had some time alone in our home. It was such a pleasure just to have some quiet time. Once we moved Michelle to her new addition at the back of the house, we had more privacy, but there was still always someone with us at all times. Larry and I had made it a point to go out to dinner together every Friday night just so that we could have some time together—just the two of us.

I still was experiencing "survivor's guilt." It was very difficult for me to go out socially and enjoy myself, while my daughter was at home without a family member. Work was my escape. It gave me the opportunity to have a break from caring for Michelle without feeling guilty. In addition, because I worked in health-care ethics, it also enabled me to continue working for Michelle and other brain-injured individuals without feeling that I was abandoning her by leaving the house. It was still very difficult to be with my friends and relatives who were helping their daughters prepare for their weddings.

We also added some other therapies to her regiment. My friend, Delia's daughter, Liz, was studying to be an art therapist at a local college, and I asked her whether she would be interested in working with Michelle. Liz agreed and began to come to our house one day a week to do art with Michelle. Michelle loved it, and told us that it was the only time that she felt that she could be creative. At first, she could only paint small areas, but as time went by she became more adept.

One day Liz was working with Michelle, and I was in the living room listening to their conversation. Michelle had made a clay man, which fell on the floor and broke. Liz said, "Oh, Michelle, what happened?" Michelle responded, "The man was hit by a car." Now both Liz and I listened very intently. Liz next said, "And then what happened." "An ambulance came and took the man to the hospital." "And then what?" "The man slept for a very long time." "Michelle, how does that make you feel? Does that make you feel sad?" Michelle's response was, "Why should that make me feel sad. It's only a clay man."

Eventually Liz had to leave us, but she recommended that one of her fellow students, Naomi, begin to work with Michelle. Naomi was wonderful also, and with Naomi's help, Michelle blossomed, now painting entire canvases. She also does many creative projects and has made some gifts.

We had also tried to have Michelle work with computers. During her first year at home we had taken her to a local center that worked with persons with disabilities. They had a well- equipped computer room with many different kinds of special equipment, but the program they attempted to set up for Michelle was unsuccessful. Then we found an individual who worked at one of the hospitals in New York City. She came to our home several times to work with Michelle, but that too did not work out. One of Michelle's problems was the ataxia that she had in her arms and hands. They shook a great deal, which made it hard to hit a computer key only once. She would hit it many times. We had ordered a special keyboard that had a cover with holes over the keys and the goal was to have her use a pencil to hit the key through the hole. Fortunately, her language center was intact and she had already known how to use a computer before her accident, so those skills were in place and did not need to be learned.

Finally, on the recommendation of another mother of a son who had TBI, I found a neuropsychologist who worked with computers and who came to the home. This was exactly what I had been looking for. Dr. Rosamond Gianutsos began working with Michelle on a weekly basis. Our goal was to have Michelle learn to use the computer and then learn to use it as a tool to help her with other functions. We began by ordering a special keyboard with larger letters. Her mouse was a joystick with a large yellow ball on the end. The computer also had filter keys, which delay typing, so that if you hit a key successively it will record the letter only once. Her computer also spoke and repeated every letter after she typed it and every word after it was completed. In the beginning, Michelle typed very slowly, but she typed.

Dr. Gianutsos set up many programs on her computer. Most of these focused on improving her memory. Michelle would view three words, and then they would disappear and she would have to type what she just saw. There were also several games. Mah-jongg became her favorite, and she would play this game for hours. The computer gave her a sense of freedom. She could play these games by herself.

As she became more proficient at the basic tasks, she moved on to more difficult programs. Soon she began to make entries into a daily diary. She also began to read and answer her own e-mail. At first this was cumbersome because she would be very repetitive and focus on her talking computer. Everyone got an e-mail that said. "I am typing this on a computer that repeats the letters after I say them."

Eventually, however, we were able to remove the talking component from the computer as well as the filter keys. She also progressed to using a regular mouse. The games that she played became more complicated. She liked playing Wheel of Fortune and guessing words. She was also able to play Set, which was her favorite game before the accident. This game required a great deal of mental stamina. In addition, she played Scattegories, and although someone else needed to type the words because she could not type rapidly, she knew the answers very quickly. Her favorite games, which she could play totally by herself, were Mah-Jongg and Bejeweled. The day-to-day progress seemed very slow, but when one looked back on where she had begun, it was amazing to see how far she had come.

Michelle even came up with mnemonic devices and codes to help her remember things. For example, when we had hired a new aide, Janetta, whose last name started with a "b," Michelle referred to her as "her brown nurse." She was using the "b" in Janetta's last name and the color of Janetta's skin to help her remember Janetta. One day, I asked Michelle if Janetta was brown because her last name started with "b," then why was she (Michelle) white. She responded in an instant, "If you take the first letter of my name and turn it upside down it's a "w." She would always add that she hoped we didn't think that she was racist, but we all knew that she was devising memory tools.

I was thrilled to have so many people from so many different backgrounds working with Michelle. As we added new nurses and new therapists, many different parts of the world were represented. Our house was like a little United Nations. There was Boris from Siberia, Guylourdes from Haiti (with whom Michelle spoke French), Glory from Panama, Janetta from Antigua, Aneta from Poland, Louis from Colombia, Evelyn, Lalita, and Leala from Guyana, Dr. Ofir from Israel. We had stumbled upon such a richly diverse staff, but I came to understand over and over again how important diversity was in healing brain injury. Different accents, different colors, different physiques provoked different memories. Michelle had always loved diversity and now she had a way of connecting someone new on staff to someone in her past. It was usually through some elaborate configuration of letters.

A turning point came for us at one of Michelle's visits to her neurologist, Dr. Wirkowski. As I was describing Michelle's bad behavior to the doctor, she asked whether I would be willing to try the drug, Effexor. Effexor is for depression, and Michelle was not depressed. Everyone thought that she should be, and she was tested several times for depression, but she was not. Nevertheless, Dr. Wirkowski said that she had had some success with this drug in other TBI patients to help control their behavior. I remembered what it had been like when we tried Provigil, so I was not excited about testing a new drug, but we had all endured over a year of terrible behavior, and behavior modification therapy was not working. Using drugs posed such an ethical dilemma for me. I did not want to drug Michelle simply to control her, and yet her quality of life and our quality of life had become severely diminished because of her behavior.

I agreed to try the drug. It was amazing. After the first small dosage of 37.5 milligrams, someone knocked on the door and Michelle said, "Come in," instead of doing her usual kicking and screaming in reaction to a knock on the door. Michelle's behavior continued to improve. It was not perfect, and there were still some flare-ups, but we were again able to take her out in public.

She began to go to church with us on Sundays, we took her to movies and plays, and were also able to take her to restaurants to eat. She still needed to have her mind engaged or she would yell that she wanted to go home. In restaurants, for example, as soon as she was finished eating she'd be ready to leave. The movies and plays needed to be light with lots of humor and action. She had difficulty following a plot. Nevertheless, this was a big improvement over her behavior in the past year.

As she forged her new identity, there were many humorous moments as well. She still had a piercing intellect, a quick wit, and the ability to express herself. But these attributes were often accompanied by behavior that was more appropriate of a two-year-old. For example, because Michelle always loved young children and wanted to be a teacher some day, I had arranged for her to work with the children in our parish church. Every Sunday, during the Mass the children are dismissed and go to the back of the church where someone teaches them about the readings of the day. I thought Michelle would be able to help teach the children because she still remembered her religion lessons, and I also thought that it would be good to have the children become comfortable with someone in a wheelchair.

Several weeks before Easter, I had helped Michelle to prepare a lesson for the children. The central theme was that Jesus loves us all, including people in wheelchairs.

Michelle told this to the children, and immediately their hands went up. One little girl told Michelle that she had once seen a dog on *Animal Planet* that had three legs. Another little boy said he had seen a sheep on *Animal Planet* that had six legs, and finally a girl added that she had seen a dog in the local park that had three legs. Michelle raised her hand, and I thought that she was going to pull everything together and explain that sitting in a wheelchair was not exactly the same as having three legs. Instead, she asked, "What channel is *Animal Planet* on?" But she connected with the children. They were all eager to tell her the time and the channel.

Helping Michelle regain an identity was very difficult. I wanted to be true to whom she was, while at the same time help her to become all she might be. Michelle was very content living in the moment. She had all her needs met, experienced love, and was not in pain. Many times she rebelled when she was in therapy. I often wondered whether I was doing the right thing by working diligently to pull her back into our world.

Clara Claiborne Park, the mother of an autistic child, Jessy, asks in her book, *Exiting Nirvana*, (Little, Brown and Company, 2001), whether it is right to lead her daughter out of what she calls Nirvana into the uncertain world of humans. Oliver Sacks says in the forward of that book that this is something we all need to do – move from some kind of primal Eden into a world of uncertainty and risk. Parks agrees. She recognizes that the human world is not Nirvana. I felt that I had to ask similar questions about Michelle's identity and the world she would want to inhabit.

I took my cues from Michelle. Because I had faced her death, I was not caught up in not being able to let her go, desperately clinging to the hope of a specific outcome. I could step back and observe. Michelle had lived and emerged from the coma, and we had simply stood by her and attempted to remove any obstacles to her recovery. Then I observed how hard Michelle had worked in therapy and how great her love for life was. Unlike Park's daughter, who knew no other world than an autistic world, Michelle had experienced a world that was not Nirvana. As long as she continued to push herself, I knew that the world that she wished to reenter was the world that she had known. Now that she can speak, she informs everyone that what she wants to do more than anything is to walk. When I asked her why, she responded that once she could walk, she could leave and I took this as a sign that she wished to regain her independence, and I would help her do so. Still, I knew Michelle's future was uncertain. I did not know whether Michelle would ever be independent. I suspected that the answer was that she would not be, but on the other hand I had also suspected that she would die and that she would not awaken. She was constantly proving everyone wrong.

I continued to deal with therapists who would periodically tell me that Michelle had plateaued and that we should discontinue therapy. At this point, we were doing mostly self-pay for our therapies, so it was not as though these therapists needed to justify their work to insurance companies or Medicaid. I began to question continued treatment for Michelle as well. Was I providing futile treatment for my daughter? Was I using scarce resources on someone who had no possibility of improving as a result of this treatment? Should I be pushing Michelle into so much therapy when she seemed to be very content to sit by her computer and play mah-jongg all day? Was I an unreasonable, overbearing mother who simply liked to be in control? I think health-care professionals often thought this, and I needed to honestly ask myself these questions.

Yet, we continued to see progress – although it was slow and uneven. Michelle had come a long way from where she was when we first brought her home. When health-care professionals were in charge in the institutions, they over-drugged her, caused her to get infections, and often ignored her. Since she had been home, she had not had one infection, began to eat by mouth, responded to her surroundings, began to speak, even began to correspond through e-mail, and told us every day that she knew that she was loved. There was a great deal of laughter in our home, and Michelle's wit was as quick as it had always been. Yes, sometimes she came out with things that were inappropriate, but very often she was right on target. So I continued to do what Larry and Michelle had once told me my PhD had trained me to do – that was research and fight, research and fight. But it was exhausting.

Following the advice of Michelle's physical therapist, Christine, we began another therapy for Michelle – therapeutic horseback riding. We looked into several programs and tried one that did not work out and then found Pal-o-Mine. This was a wonderful program. It was specifically set up for persons with disabilities. At first, Michelle needed lots of help because it was difficult for her to even sit on the horse and keep her balance. Four people worked with her. Two people walked with her, one on each side of her, one person led the horse, and a physical therapist walked in front giving her directions. She started the program receiving short lessons during which she would spend most of her time just getting comfortable in the saddle; these turned into sessions in which she rode out on the trails. She loved the horse she rode, named Yankee, even though she kept telling the therapists that she would prefer to ride a horse named Met, in order to be faithful to her father's baseball allegiance.

Another therapy that we began the summer after Michelle had her feeding tube removed was swimming. Aunt Noreen lived around the corner from us and had a swimming pool. Our case manager found a male physical therapist named Doug, who was willing to go to Aunt Noreen's pool twice a week and help Michelle with swimming. Doug was not only a talented physical therapist but also quite good looking, and Michelle loved working with him. In the beginning, it was difficult to have Michelle walk down the three steps into the pool but eventually she got to the point where she would even put her head under water and blow bubbles. When she was in the pool with us and without Doug, she wore a plastic tube to keep her floating on the surface. She loved the freedom of being able to go wherever she wanted to in the water. When she was with Doug, she would often work with only a small foam board strapped to her back. Her right side was still much weaker than her left side so her swimming was uneven but she was able to do many things in the pool that she was not able to do outside the pool.

Eventually, we added two other therapies. I had read a book about biofeedback and how it helped individuals with certain conditions. I thought it might help Michelle to focus better and concentrate. One of the therapists mentioned in the book worked at a hospital close to our home, and I contacted him. He did an initial evaluation and then began to work with Michelle on a weekly basis. In a short time, his program was discontinued and he lived too far away to take Michelle to his other office, but he recommended another psychologist who worked with biofeedback who lived close by. We contacted Dr. Malone, and Michelle began to work with him.

It was fascinating to watch Michelle in therapy. Three electrodes were attached to her head. The positioning varied depending on what skill the therapy was focusing on. Michelle then watched a computer screen and performed an activity using her brain waves. For example, one program had a maze with a little fish. Michelle needed "to think" the fish through the maze. Every fish movement was accompanied by the sound of a fish moving through the water. There were many other programs, and Michelle worked very hard. The therapists could not tell Michelle what to do, other than relax. Michelle needed to figure out what was required on her own. She needed to remember the subjective feeling of what worked and then reapply it. Whenever it came to memory exercises, I had observed that if there was an affective dimension attached to the object, Michelle's memory was better. She remembered children's and animals' names better than adults' names.

We also added Reiki. I knew we needed something to help Michelle relax, and I thought Reiki might be helpful. Reiki works with energy fields and can be very healing and soothing. Dorinne, a Reiki master, came to our home once a week in the evening and did Reiki with Michelle. There was an immediate bond between the two of them. Like so many others, Dorinne told me that there was something special about Michelle, something very spiritual. Since Cook County Hospital, I had heard people tell me this. What it was exactly I don't know, but I did see how Michelle touched certain people.

Eventually we also hired Maria, who replaced Dr. Ofir for feldenkrais, and Pam, who worked in music therapy.

We also had Boris who did a more unconventional type of music therapy. Our goal was to attempt to reach every part of Michelle's brain.

Again we saw the importance of relationships. When individuals cannot initiate on their own or determine what is in their best interests, they need others to do this for them. We are never formed totally on our own but in a community. We needed to use everything we had learned throughout this process to help her form her new identity. Our bonds to her and our recognition that she was a gift in our lives are what kept us committed. We needed to appreciate and recognize that each brain is different and that there is a great deal of ambiguity involved in her progress. It is not steady improvement but involves both advances and setbacks. Slow healing was also part of the process.

Michelle's brain, the seat of her personhood, was injured, and her identity was fractured. Her core identity was still intact, but she needed help to reestablish her autobiographical identity. The best people to be involved in this process were members of her family, the same people who had helped her form her former identity. But this required large amounts of time and resources. It also suggested a new model of providing health care – a model that took long-term care as seriously as acute care – a model that suggested a redistribution of resources that included nursing and therapy as well as MRI and CAT scans. It also suggested a change of setting, away from an institutional milieu to the patient's home, which could occur only if the resources supported it, otherwise, it would be too overwhelming for a family to take on this responsibility.

Michelle is slowly forming her new identity. Her fractured pieces are beginning to coalesce. We still see the old Michelle but with new talents. Before the accident, everything came easily to Michelle; now she needs to work very hard in everything that she does. Every part of her needs to be reformed, not just her cognitive skills, but her walking, her talking, her motor skills.

The most difficult part to restructure is her social life. Her friends have moved on, as expected, but she has little opportunity to make new friends. She goes to day programs twice a week where she meets other individuals with brain injuries, but this is not the same as having friends with whom she can go out and reenter the social world. Part of this is forgetfulness on the part of her former friends but part of it also is that Michelle is unable to hold up her part of the relationship. Friendships rely on mutuality and a relationship with Michelle requires different skills than is usually expected from a friendship. At first glance, it appears that someone who developed a friendship with Michelle would do all the giving, but for those of us who have lived and cared for her these past ten years, we know that we too have changed and have been taught a great deal by Michelle. We are better persons because of her.

In *Tuesdays with Morrie*, Morrie states that what he feared the most was getting to the point where he could no longer wipe his behind. But I learned that worse than that was that when that day came there would no one there to wipe it for you. Whether we are disabled or not, we need each other.

Again a quote on her wall inspired us: "Never tell a young person that anything cannot be done. God may have been waiting centuries for someone ignorant enough of the impossible to do that very thing." With our help we hoped that Michelle would accomplish the impossible. After several years at home, we had created a new life for Michelle. She usually had about five or six hours of therapy a day. Her day often began with one of her occupational therapists, Tricia or Jessica, coming to help her get dressed and make her breakfast. Then she would go out to physical therapy or speech therapy or biofeedback. She'd come home for lunch and then have art, vision, or cognitive therapy. On weekends, she'd have music therapy, feldenkrais, and go horseback riding. We also added massage therapy. Two days a week she would go to a day program and have therapy there as well as have the opportunity to socialize. Between therapies she would play games on her computer, answer her e-mail, or go out to movies, plays, etc.

I worked with Michelle's therapists as a team member. We were all involved in a grand experiment. As Dr. O'Dell once said to me when I questioned him about a medication, "Truthfully, Mrs. Martone, this far post-injury, we really don't know." I knew that this was the case. Fifteen years ago, Michelle would have died from her injuries. Medicine was now at the point where it knew how to save her life. Medicine had also determined how to establish high-quality acute-care facilities to help those with TBI. But if one did not make a rapid recovery in these institutions, very few professionals knew what to do next, other than to recommend that the patient be sent to a nursing home, which did not provide rehabilitation and where recovery then became almost impossible.

Although our therapists and nurses were a patchwork team, individuals whom I had found and whom I coordinated, things seemed to be working. Once a year, around the Christmas holidays, we would have a thank-you party, where the individual therapists, physicians, and nurses got to meet each other and discuss Michelle's progress. Everything focused on Michelle and how we might help her improve.

After nine years at home, we had made a great deal of progress. Michelle walks with a walker, although her balance is still a major issue. She feeds herself, dresses herself, answers her own e-mail, speaks in full, under-standable sentences, and initiates conversation. Her memory is still an issue but continues to improve. She is able to go out to movies, theater, horseback riding, and family parties. She is an integral part of our family. When we built her addition to our home in the back of the house, I was afraid that she would be shunted away from the heart of the family, but I discovered that all of us moved to the back with her. Everyone simply began using the back door.

As a family, our lives continued also. Two of our sons, Tim and Larry, married, and we are lucky to have two won-derful daughters-in-law, Melissa and Pauline. Larry and Pauline soon gave birth to a beautiful daughter, Alexis Elizabeth who also became part of our lives and grew up knowing her Aunt Michelle. Unlike most little children, Alexis was not afraid of individuals in wheelchairs or who were a little different from others. Alexis loved sharing her food with Michelle, climbing into her wheelchair, and playing ball with Michelle. Several years later Alexis had a sister, Summer. All three of our sons continue to visit regularly with their sister and to take her out on adven-tures. Melissa, Pauline, Alexis, and Summer also became integral parts of her life.

Larry semi-retired, and helped with the driving to therapy, the finances, the judge's reports, and all the paperwork. Larry and I began to take vacations, although, in the beginning, we traveled separately. It seemed that there was always a crisis, such as the electric bed breaking while in the upright position, the toilet bowl cracking and water running all over the floor, the computer crashing, the electric door of the van not closing, someone calling in sick or quitting. The only way I felt that I could go away and fully relax was if Larry was home and in charge. Besides, he was able to go on his baseball tours and country music trips – things I had no desire to do – while I went to the spa and Europe. Lately, however, our staff has coalesced and become more reliable and Larry and I have been able to go away together.

This is not the life that we had envisioned for ourselves, but it is a good life. We are still together as a family, and we have a daughter who tells us every day how much she loves us.

A quote from the *Tao of Pooh* probably best summarizes the culmination of these past years: "The Athletic sort of Backson – one of the many common varieties – is concerned with physical fitness, he says. But for some reason, he sees it as something that has to be pounded in from the outside, rather than built up from the inside. Therefore, he confuses exercise with work. He works when he works, works when he exercises, and, more often than not, works when he plays. Work, work, work. All work and no play makes Backson a dull boy. Kept up for long enough, it makes him dead, too."

Exhausted—that would be the best way to describe how I've felt since Michelle's accident. First there was the emotional exhaustion of sitting by her bedside for hours and going through the roller-coaster ride of surgeries, infections, and near deaths. Then there was the constant watchfulness over her rehabilitation, waiting for the next family meeting where we would be told that Michelle was not meeting the facility's expectations and that we would have to leave. There were also the relapses of pneumonia, urinary track infections, the surprise seizures, as well as the many medication issues. In addition to these, there were the draining days when Michelle would perform poorly in therapy or the days when her behavior was so bad and the screaming so loud and consistent that I thought I would lose my mind.

In addition to the emotional exhaustion there was also the physical exhaustion. There were days in Chicago when I could barely get out of bed, but I knew that my daughter needed me so I did. There was the driving back and forth to New Jersey and eastern Long Island as well as the toting of laundry and other supplies. There were the sixteen ambulance rides that I went on with her. When we brought her home, there was cooking, cleaning, changing bed linens, organizing staff, hiring and firing staff, sorting through paperwork, the staying on top of payroll, and much negotiating.

All of this took a toll on me physically. Frequently, Michelle's wheelchair rolled over my foot (once it fractured my toe). When she lost her balance, we would often bump heads, and when she started to walk with a walker, I developed bursitis in my left shoulder, which eventually turned into a frozen shoulder. During this time, I also had both knees replaced, breast cancer surgery and radiation treatment, and my gall bladder removed. But I never missed a day of work except when I had emergency gall bladder surgery. Through all of this, I also managed to complete my preparation for and succeed in attaining tenure.

One advantage I gained was learning how to become totally focused. I was able to block out the day-to-day nonsense, and focus on what needed to be done. I began to concentrate my research on brain injury, rehabilitation, chronic care, and disability. I read and published widely in this area. During the summer of 2002, I received an NEH (National Endowment for the Humanities) grant to participate in a summer seminar entitled, "Justice, Equality, and the Challenge of Disability," and worked with two senior scholars in this area, Anita Silvers and Eva Kittay. Most recently, I received a six-month fellowship to work at Weill Cornell Medical College and the Hospital for Special Surgery on disability ethics. In addition to my teaching and committee activities at St. John's, I am a fellow in the Vincentian Center for Church and Society, where my work focuses on just distribution of health-care resources. Also, since 2004, I have been one of the Holy See representatives to the United Nations on women's issues.

What drives me? Why do I continually push myself when my body is telling me to slow down? Am I like the Bisy Backson in the *Tao of Pooh*, about whom it is said, "if you want to be healthy, relaxed, and contented, just watch what a Bisy Backson does and then do the opposite." Am I driving myself to extinction? I know too that I could be a better wife, a better mother to my other children, a better grandmother, and yet I lie in bed at night wondering what else I might do to help Michelle. Why am I so obsessed with her recovery? I had been ready to accept her death, but I am not willing to allow her to languish in front of a computer or a television (which she hardly ever watches). I am driven, and I drive her.

The best way of explaining why I function the way I do now is that I went over the waterfall also. So did my entire family. But while Michelle entered unconsciousness as she went over and the rest of the family came down in lifeboats, I was put in charge of gathering the pieces and putting them back together again. Although the accident happened to Michelle, in a way it is more my experience than hers because she has no memory of it or the months following it. The hospitals and rehabilitation facilities, years of therapy and hard work to improve her condition, reuniting with friends and family, formed my memory, not Michelle's. I was more intent on fighting for her survival than she was. She just survived, but I had to work to make it happen.

But was I working too hard? Our best moments together were when I had no expectations of her, and we just enjoyed each other's company. But I wasn't working just for her. Throughout this process I had seen first hand the injustices built into our health-care system. Those without health-care insurance received acute care through hospital emergency rooms, but after that it became very difficult to access services. The services that were available were in many cases sub-standard with little continuity of care. In a subsequent trip to Chicago I went back to Cook County Hospital and encountered the woman who ran the elevator whose daughter had been in the ICU with Michelle. I asked her how her daughter was and she responded, "She passed." She had died in the county rehab facility from choking on her mucus.

Even for people who had insurance, once they endured a catastrophic illness, they were often reduced to poverty. The only reason we could care for Michelle the way we did was because we had a large legal settlement. Even as an upper-middle-class family, Michelle's illness and recovery would have drained all our resources. Almost all of her therapies are self-pay. Insurance coverage stopped a long time ago.

Most families who are caring for brain-injured individuals not only don't have the resources, but also don't have the time to advocate for their loved ones. Care giving involves large amounts of time. We were able to hire caregivers so that I could return to work. Also, the fact that I work in health-care ethics opened many doors for me that would not be open to other mothers.

I need to do what I am doing, not only for Michelle, but also for other persons who are brain injured as well as their families. It is critical that I do this now, when many members of our armed forces are returning from Iraq and Afghanistan severely injured. These are young men and women who have given the best years of their lives to serve our country and who are returned in the dead of night and transported to military hospitals where we, the public, do not see the devastation that war has had on them and their families. The only way I know to return the gifts that we have been given is to become the voice of those who have no voice or no time to express their voice.

We, as a society, need to embrace persons with brain injuries. Many individuals and communities who were present to us in the acute care phase faded away when they recognized that their relationship needed to be readjusted. Living in solidarity with someone who is vulnerable can make you vulnerable as well. Not everyone is ready for this. But persons with brain injuries must be protected against losing their dignity and having others consider them less than human. I cannot sit quietly and watch as society ignores these individuals and shunts them into institutions where they are forgotten. We take Michelle everywhere. Society needs to see her. I don't care if others are embarrassed or uncomfortable when they are around her. In her, all of our humanity is present. She forces us to come face to face with our vulnerabilities and weaknesses. She reminds us that we too will probably some day become disabled. It is part of the human condition.

Jean Vanier, the founder of L'Arche Communities for persons with cognitive disability, highlights in his book, *Becoming Human* (Anansi 1998) how we create barriers to protect our vulnerability and Eric Goffman, author of the seminal book, *Stigma* (Simon and Schuster, 1963) describes these barriers as stigma. Stigma, he states, "does not so much represent a set of concrete individuals who can be separated into two piles, the stigmatized and the normal, as a pervasive two-role social process in which every individual participates in both roles, at least in some connections and in some phases of life. The normal and the stigmatized are not persons but perspectives." (pp. 137-138) In reality then, in marginalizing persons with disabilities we are marginalizing those parts of ourselves that represent a loss of control, autonomy, and self-government. Persons with disabilities are reminders that everything cannot be controlled by our will and that life is sometimes unpredictable and chaotic. In a world where it is important to have power and social status, aligning ourselves with persons with disabilities diminishes us.

Yet many authors remind us that being human means more than self-sufficiency and autonomy. The noted philosopher, Alasdair MacIntyre reminds us that acknowledgment of dependence is the key to independence. Eva Kittay, a feminist philosopher, reminds us that we are all dependent and our fates hang on those of others. The goal of life is to increase the level of joy one can experience. Thomas Reynolds, in *Vulnerable Communities* (Brazos Press 2008) states that the basic question of human existence is whether there is a welcome at the heart of things. And Hans Reinders in *Receiving the Gift of Friendship* (William B. Eerdmans, 2008) questions why it is assumed that the only friends that persons with disabilities have should be other persons with disabilities.

For me, the fear of abandonment and marginalization has been my constant companion throughout our journey. There is still much work to be done. This is why I write and why I work to the point of exhaustion. I am determined to have Michelle, and our family, remain an integral part of society. I want to help build sustainable communities, communities that do not ignore those members who are not self-sufficient; communities where those who are able, care for those who need care; communities where individuals stop running away from their fears but face them; communities where we all recognize that it is only in the faces of others that we are able to see the face of God.

Deus Caritas Est. That is what I had read and been told before I began this journey. God is love is what I find as I continue.

8480414R0

Made in the USA
Lexington, KY
06 February 2011